HOME-BASED WALL PILATES FOR BEGINNERS, SENIORS

EXERCISES TO INCREASE BALANCE, IMPROVE
POSTURE, FLEXIBILITY, AND REINFORCE STABILITY
FOR VISIBLE BODY TRANSFORMATION IN AS LITTLE
AS 29-DAYS

SEBASTIAN CASTELLANOS

CONTENTS

INTRODUCTION

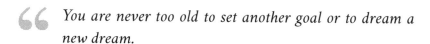 *You are never too old to set another goal or to dream a new dream.*

— LES BROWN

In a world where age is often misconstrued as a limitation, let me introduce you to Vera Teachout, a spirited 65-year-old, and Cheri Hunt, a determined 73-year-old, both blazing trails in the realm of senior fitness (Kouvo, 2021). Not only are they rewriting the narrative, but they're also dispelling myths with each weight they lift, every stride they take, and every beat of their heart.

These remarkable women have made exercise a cornerstone of their retired lives, defying societal norms that suggest other-wise. Vera and Cheri, with their silver-streaked hair and unyielding determination, are living proof that age is no barrier to vitality. Their journey began with the "Forever Fit" program, a beacon for mature individuals seeking to embrace invigorating workouts in a warm and encouraging setting.

Vera's story began a few years ago when she noticed her golf swing losing its vigor and household chores leaving her weary. Undeterred, she stepped into the gym, greeted by peers in her age group and a staff that welcomed her with open arms. There, she discovered a sanctuary free of judgment, focused solely on personal progress rather than competition.

As the days passed, Vera's golf swing roared back to life, paralleled only by her newfound confidence in everyday tasks. Simple acts like unloading groceries and stepping out of the car became second nature once more. And when the pandemic reared its head, the gym's unwavering support persisted, offering virtual training and stringent safety measures for those seeking refuge in their fitness journey.

In sunny Florida, Cheri's story unfolded, marked by a pivotal moment when a pair of snug pants signaled the need for change. Once 40 pounds heavier and struggling to move, Cheri's determination led her back to regular exercise. Her transformation wasn't just physical; it was a testament to the power of dedication and self-resilience. Through the guidance of caring coaches and her favorite leg press machine, Cheri's strength, balance, and overall well-being soared to new heights (Kouvo, 2021).

These women stand as living testaments to the incredible transformations awaiting anyone, at any age, who dares to take the first step. Joining the right gym or studio and committing to a consistent fitness routine—are the keys to a vibrant, empowered life, regardless of the number of candles on your birthday cake.

Vera and Cheri's inspiring stories aren't just anecdotes—they resonate with millions of older adults who grapple with mobility challenges every day. In fact, statistics reveal a startling truth: Approximately 36 million falls occur among older adults annually, tragically leading to over 32,000 fatalities (CDC, 2020). These numbers underscore the urgency of addressing the issue.

Consider this: Each year, a staggering 3 million older adults find themselves in emergency departments due to fall-related injuries. One out of every five falls results in severe consequences, ranging from fractured bones to head trauma (CDC, 2020). The impact of these incidents reverberates far beyond the immediate physical toll—they can shake the very foundation of one's confidence and independence.

The gravity of these statistics paints a vivid picture of the risks older individuals face. However, it also underscores the power of proactive measures. Vera and Cheri's commitment to regular exercise and strength-building not only defies stereotypes but also serves as a beacon of hope for those seeking to reclaim their mobility, confidence, and quality of life.

I understand the challenges you might be facing. For many, the struggle with mobility is more than just a physical hurdle—it's a daily battle against the limitations that age can impose. The ache in your joints, the stiffness in your muscles, and that nagging back pain can become constant companions, sapping not only your physical vitality but also your enthusiasm for the activities that once brought you joy.

Perhaps, like Vera, you've noticed a decline in your once-effortless routines. Maybe it's those once-enjoyable walks with loved ones that have become a source of discomfort or the realization that specific household tasks now leave you fatigued and sore. It's in these moments of realization that a spark of determination often ignites—the catalyst that propels you toward seeking a solution.

For Cheri, it was the tight fit of a pair of pants that served as her wake-up call. The mirror offered a candid reflection of the changes she had undergone, and it was a moment of clarity that demanded action. Her journey from that pivotal moment is a testament to the transformative power of commitment and perseverance.

I know that you, like Vera and Cheri, yearn for more than just a return to daily functionality. You desire the freedom to move without restraint, to engage in activities that bring you fulfillment, and to revel in the simple pleasures that life has to offer.

By diving into this book, you're embarking on a transformative journey that promises an array of valuable benefits tailored precisely for individuals like you.

Better health: Discover exercises and techniques that are specifically curated to enhance your physical well-being. Through the practice of Wall Pilates, you'll forge a stronger, more flexible body, allowing you to navigate your daily activities with newfound ease.

Mental clarity: It's not just about the body; this book places equal emphasis on nurturing your mental health. By incorporating mindfulness techniques, you'll journey toward reduced stress levels and a sharper, clearer mind. Say goodbye to mental fog and embrace a renewed sense of focus and clarity.

Save money: Say "farewell" to costly gym memberships and specialized equipment. With a focus on Wall Pilates exercises that can be seamlessly integrated into your home routine, you'll find that achieving your fitness goals can be both convenient and affordable.

Easy to follow: Designed with beginners and seniors in mind, this book ensures that the exercises are presented in a clear, step-by-step manner. Even if you're new to Pilates or the fitness world, you'll find the instructions easy to grasp and execute, paving the way for a seamless and enjoyable experience.

Community and support: In your pursuit of a healthier, more vibrant you, this book doesn't just stop at exercises. It guides you toward a community of like-minded individuals, providing the invaluable support and motivation you may need along the way. Together, you'll forge a path toward wellness bolstered by the strength of a united community.

Over the next 29 days, you're about to embark on a transformative journey toward better health, increased flexibility, and enhanced mental clarity. This book is your steadfast companion, designed with your unique needs in mind, whether you're a beginner or a seasoned senior seeking to rejuvenate your well-being.

Every day of this program will introduce you to thoughtfully selected Wall Pilates exercises, complemented by mindfulness techniques designed to enhance not only your physical strength but also your mental well-being. You'll discover that these exercises are not only highly effective but also incredibly accessible, utilizing common items like chairs and towels as your instruments of transformation. This approach ensures that you can seamlessly integrate these practices into your daily routine, leading to a holistic improvement in both body and mind.

After completing this 29-day journey, you will have not only established a solid foundation of beneficial Wall Pilates habits but also witnessed the remarkable positive effects it can bring to your life. Enhanced balance, greater flexibility, decreased stress, and heightened mental clarity will accompany you on this transformative journey towards a revitalized and improved version of yourself.

This journey extends far beyond mere physical transformation. It's a profound endeavor aimed at regaining control, reshaping the narrative of aging, and adopting a lifestyle that empowers you to embrace life's fullest potential. Let's embark on this journey together and uncover the extraordinary capabilities within you. Hand in hand, we'll carve out a path leading to a more vibrant, healthier, and ultimately happier version of yourself.

1

THE FOUNDATIONS OF WALL PILATES

Allow me to introduce you to Heather Andersen, a trailblazer in the world of Pilates. Heather's journey began in high school, where she discovered Pilates as a vital component of her training as a pre-professional ballet dancer. Her passion for this transformative practice only grew, leading her to complete rigorous certifications in both mat Pilates and gyrotonic techniques. Heather's quest for deeper knowledge took her to the renowned Irene Dowd, an anatomy expert at The Juilliard School (Andersen, 2023).

Armed with a wealth of experience and a profound under-standing of the human body, Heather founded New York Pilates with a mission to revolutionize the Pilates experience. Her approach is all about making Pilates accessible, enjoyable, and most importantly, empowering. Through her unique perspective, informed by diverse training backgrounds and years of dedicated teaching, Heather has paved the way for a new era in Pilates.

Today, New York Pilates has certified over 200 exceptional instructors, each carrying forth Heather's vision to studios and gyms worldwide (Andersen, 2023). The impact of Heather's work transcends mere workouts and repetitions; it's about teaching people how to effect profound changes, not just in their bodies but in their lives. The story of Heather Andersen serves as an inspiring testament to the transformative power of Pilates, and it's the foundation upon which we'll build your Pilates journey in the pages ahead.

UNDERSTANDING WALL PILATES: PRINCIPLES AND BENEFITS

Wall Pilates is a dynamic and highly effective form of exercise that combines the principles of traditional Pilates with the support and resistance provided by a wall. It offers a unique approach to body conditioning, focusing on strength, flexibility, balance, and alignment. This innovative method harnesses the stability of a wall to enhance the effectiveness of each movement, allowing for a deeper engagement of muscles and a more controlled range of motion.

At its core, Wall Pilates encourages a mind-body connection, emphasizing precise movements and controlled breathing patterns. By incorporating the wall into exercises, practitioners are provided with an additional source of support, allowing them to perform movements with greater stability and confidence. This not only aids in building core strength but also facilitates a heightened awareness of posture and alignment.

Wall Pilates is a versatile practice that can be tailored to individual needs and abilities. Whether you're a beginner or have some prior experience with Pilates, the principles remain consistent. It's about fostering a harmonious relationship between your body and the wall, allowing you to tap into your full potential for physical well-being.

Wall Pilates, an innovative variation of the traditional Pilates method, draws its roots from the rich history of Pilates itself. Developed by Joseph Pilates in the early 20th century, Pilates was initially known as "contrology." Joseph Pilates was a German-born fitness enthusiast who dedicated his life to understanding the intricate connection between the mind and body (Pilates Foundation, 2020).

His unique approach to exercise was heavily influenced by his background in gymnastics, yoga, and martial arts. During World War I, Joseph Pilates worked as a nurse, rehabilitating wounded soldiers. It was here that he began to refine his techniques, utilizing springs attached to hospital beds to facilitate resistance-based exercises.

After the war, Pilates immigrated to the United States and set up a studio in New York City. There, he continued to develop and refine his exercise method, emphasizing the importance of core strength, flexibility, and controlled movements. His method garnered a loyal following among dancers, athletes, and individuals seeking a holistic approach to fitness (Pilates Foundation, 2020).

Over time, Pilates' method evolved, with practitioners incorporating various props and equipment to enhance the exercises. This evolution gave rise to Wall Pilates, a dynamic adaptation that utilizes the support and resistance of a wall to further engage muscles and refine movements.

Today, Wall Pilates stands as a testament to the enduring legacy of Joseph Pilates' innovative approach to fitness. It exemplifies the versatility and adaptability of the Pilates method, providing practitioners with a powerful tool to enhance their strength, flexibility, and overall well-being.

The Benefits of Wall Pilates

Wall Pilates holds the key to unlocking a rejuvenated sense of vitality and youthfulness. This innovative practice offers a host of transformative benefits that can make a profound difference in how you feel and move. Let's explore the primary advantages of embracing Wall Pilates.

Improved balance and stability: Wall Pilates engages your core muscles and emphasizes proper alignment. This translates to better stability and balance, which are crucial for preventing falls and maintaining confidence in your day-to-day activities.

Enhanced posture: By focusing on alignment and core strength, Wall Pilates helps correct postural imbalances. This leads to a more upright and aligned posture, reducing strain on your spine and muscles.

Increased flexibility and range of motion: Gentle stretches and controlled movements in Wall Pilates can gradually improve your flexibility. This newfound range of motion can make a world of difference in your everyday movements, from reaching for objects to simply turning your head with ease.

Greater core strength: Your core muscles are like the power-house of your body. Wall Pilates targets these muscles, promoting a stronger core. This not only aids in posture and balance but also supports your spine and reduces the risk of back pain.

Reduced stress and improved mental clarity: The mind-body connection in Wall Pilates incorporates mindful breathing and focused movements. This combination leads to reduced stress levels and a more transparent and focused mind. It's a holistic approach that nurtures both your physical and mental well-being.

Why Wall Pilates

As we gracefully navigate the journey of aging, prioritizing our physical well-being takes on an increasingly significant role. Among the chief concerns for seniors, the risk of falls looms large, carrying the potential of severe injuries. This is where Wall Pilates steps in as a powerful ally. By immersing yourself in this dynamic practice, you're not merely exercising; you're proactively fortifying your body against the potential hazards of imbalance and instability. Through meticulously designed movements and the support of the wall, Wall Pilates becomes a beacon of strength, empowering you to move with confidence and grace.

Moreover, the benefits extend to the very core of your being. Picture a life with improved posture—a gift that not only radiates confidence but also alleviates the discomfort and tension that often plague the back and neck, particularly in the face of age-related changes in the spine. With Wall Pilates, you're nurturing a foundation of strength and alignment that allows you to stand tall, move freely, and relish each moment with a newfound sense of vitality.

Yet, Wall Pilates doesn't stop at the physical. Its influence resonates profoundly in your daily life, enabling you to embrace a lifestyle of vigor and independence. The enhanced flexibility and core strength you'll gain aren't just assets in the studio; they're your ticket to an active, engaged existence. Whether it's joining in playtime with grandchildren, embarking on leisurely strolls through nature's beauty, or immersing yourself in cherished hobbies, Wall Pilates empowers you to revel in life's most treasured moments.

And let's not overlook the mental treasures that Wall Pilates bestows. In the midst of controlled movements and mindful breathing, you'll discover a sanctuary of calm and mental clarity. This tranquility is not only a respite from the demands of daily life but also a wellspring of enhanced cognitive function and emotional well-being. It's a priceless facet of the Wall Pilates experience, enriching your overall quality of life and illuminating the path to a more vibrant, fulfilling existence.

PREPARING YOUR SPACE: SETTING UP AT HOME AND SAFETY

Preparing your space for Wall Pilates is more than just arranging a few items—it's about setting the stage for a transformative and enriching experience. A well-prepared space ensures you have enough room to move freely without any hindrances. This allows you to fully extend your arms and legs, enabling a broader range of motion for each exercise. It also provides the mental freedom to focus solely on your practice without distractions or limitations.

Additionally, a clean and clutter-free environment minimizes the risk of accidents or injuries. By removing potential tripping hazards and ensuring proper lighting, you're creating a safe space where you can move with confidence and ease. Additionally, having a stable surface and supportive wall ensures you can perform exercises with stability and comfort.

Moreover, a well-prepared space fosters a sense of calm and focus. When your surroundings are organized and inviting, it allows you to fully immerse yourself in the practice, enhancing your mental clarity and mindfulness. This is essential for reaping the full benefits of Wall Pilates both physically and mentally.

Maybe we can word this sentence like: When your space is ready and inviting, you're more likely to stick to your practice routine. It eliminates the need for last-minute adjustments or delays, making it easier to incorporate Wall Pilates into your daily or weekly schedule. Consistency is key to experiencing lasting benefits and progress.

Selecting the Right Spot

Choosing the ideal location is pivotal for a comfortable and effective Wall Pilates practice.

Ample room for movement: It's essential to choose a location that provides you with sufficient space to move freely. This means a spot where you can fully extend your arms and legs without bumping into furniture or other objects. This unrestricted space ensures that you can perform each exercise with precision and ease, allowing for more effective practice.

Inviting atmosphere with natural light: Natural light can have a significant impact on your practice. It creates a warm and inviting atmosphere, elevating your overall experience. The presence of natural light not only enhances your mood but also allows you to better focus on your movements. If possible, position your practice area near a window to benefit from this energizing element.

Ventilation for comfort: Adequate ventilation is crucial for maintaining a comfortable practice environment. Proper airflow helps regulate temperature and prevents the space from becoming too stuffy. This ensures that you can engage in your Wall Pilates routine without discomfort or distraction, allowing you to immerse yourself in the practice fully.

Flat, unobstructed wall: The quality of the wall itself is paramount. It should be flat and free from any obstructions or protrusions that could impede your movements. This ensures that you have a stable surface to lean against, facilitating the execution of exercises. A clear wall allows for better alignment, enabling you to get the most out of each movement.

Undisturbed practice space: Select a location where you can practice without interruption. This is crucial for maintaining focus and flow during your Wall Pilates session. Choosing a spot away from high-traffic areas or areas prone to disruptions ensures that you can fully engage in the practice without external distractions.

Supportive flooring: The type of flooring beneath your practice area matters. Opt for a surface that provides adequate support and cushioning. Wood, laminate, or carpeted floors are preferable as they offer a comfortable base for your exercises. This helps absorb impact, reducing strain on your joints and ensuring a more comfortable practice.

Additional Equipment

To enhance your practice, consider investing in a few basic items. A yoga or Pilates mat provides cushioning and grip. If you're using a chair, ensure it's stable and without wheels. Resistance bands and small weights can be useful for some exercises. However, remember that Wall Pilates is designed to be accessible, so you don't need an extensive set of equipment to get started.

Prioritizing Safety

Safety is paramount in any fitness routine, and Wall Pilates is no exception. To keep your space hazard-free, clear the floor of any potential tripping hazards. Ensure there's adequate lighting, especially if you're practicing in the early morning or evening. If possible, have a phone nearby in case of emergencies. Finally, listen to your body and practice within your comfort zone to avoid overexertion or strain.

By adhering to these tips and creating a conducive environment, you're setting the stage for a safe, enjoyable, and effective Wall Pilates practice right in the comfort of your own home. Remember, the goal is to create a space that supports your journey toward improved health and well-being.

GETTING STARTED: ASSESSING FITNESS AND SETTING GOALS

Before embarking on your Wall Pilates journey, it's crucial to take stock of your current fitness level and establish clear, achievable goals. This process not only helps tailor your practice to your unique needs but also provides a roadmap for progress.

Self-Assessment of Fitness Level

Begin by honestly evaluating your current physical condition. Consider factors such as flexibility, strength, balance, and any existing health concerns. This self-assessment serves as a starting point, allowing you to track your progress over time.

Cardiovascular Endurance

Cardiovascular endurance measures your heart and lung's ability to supply oxygen-rich blood to your muscles during prolonged physical activity. To assess this, consider the following methods:

3-MINUTE STEP TEST

- Use a sturdy step or platform about 12 inches high.
- Step up and down for 3 minutes at a consistent pace.
- Measure your heart rate immediately after.
- For men between the ages of 46 and 55, a pulse rate below 93 is considered good to excellent, whereas 113 or higher is deemed fair to poor. Similarly, for women in the same age group, a pulse rate of 101 or lower is considered good to excellent, while 125 or higher is classified as fair to poor (Orenstein, 2012).

1-MILE WALK TEST

- Walk a mile as briskly as possible.
- Note the time it takes to complete the mile.
- Compare your time to age-specific norms.
- Below 14 minutes (for men) or 17 minutes (for women): Excellent
- 14-16 minutes (for men) or 17-19 minutes (for women): Good

- 17-19 minutes (for men) or 20-22 minutes (for women):
  Average
- 20-22 minutes (for men) or 23-26 minutes (for women):
  Fair
- 23 minutes or above (for men) or 27 minutes or above
  (for women): Poor

Muscular Strength and Endurance

This assesses your muscle's ability to exert force and sustain it over an extended period. Try the following tests:

PUSH-UP TEST (QUINN, 2022)

- Perform as many push-ups as possible without resting.
- Record the number of repetitions completed.

PLANK TEST (QUINN, 2022)

- Assume a plank position with forearms on the ground
  and body straight.
- Hold for as long as possible.
- Note the duration.
- Less than 10 seconds: This suggests a low level of core
  strength and endurance. Consider incorporating
  exercises to improve core stability.
- 10-20 seconds: This indicates a basic level of core
  strength. With consistent practice, you can work
  toward increasing your plank duration.

Flexibility

Flexibility evaluates your range of motion around your joints. Consider these assessments:

SIT-AND-REACH TEST

- Sit on the floor with legs extended and feet against a box or step.
- Reach forward as far as possible along a measuring line.
- Note the distance reached.
- Above +15 cm: Excellent
- +10 to +15 cm: Good
- +5 to +10 cm: Average
- 0 to +5 cm: Fair
- Below 0 cm: Poor, and this is a call to take Wall Pilates more seriously.

SHOULDER FLEXIBILITY TEST

- Stand with one hand behind your back, reaching up.
- Reach down from above with the other hand.
- Measure the distance between your hands.
- The goal is to reduce the distance between your hands.

Remember, these assessments are meant to provide a baseline understanding of your current fitness level. They should not replace a professional evaluation. If you have any existing health conditions or concerns, it's advisable to consult with a healthcare provider before starting a new exercise regimen.

Setting Achievable Goals

Setting achievable fitness goals is a crucial step toward a successful Wall Pilates practice. Here are some tips to help you set realistic and attainable goals:

Be specific and clear: Clearly define what you want to achieve with Wall Pilates. For example, instead of a vague goal like "improve flexibility," specify "increase hamstring flexibility by 2 inches."

Set measurable targets: Establish concrete metrics to track your progress. This could involve measurements, repetitions, durations, or specific achievements like holding a plank for a certain amount of time.

Consider your current fitness level: Take into account your starting point. Setting goals that are aligned with your current abilities ensures they're realistic and attainable.

Break down long-term goals: If you have a larger, long-term goal, break it down into smaller, manageable milestones. Celebrating these smaller achievements along the way provides motivation and a sense of accomplishment.

Set realistic timeframes: Be practical about the time it will take to achieve your goals. While progress is achievable, it's important to give yourself enough time to see meaningful results.

Make goals relevant to you: Your goals should align with your personal motivations and aspirations. Consider how achieving these goals will enhance your overall well-being and quality of life.

Adaptability is key: Remain flexible with your goals. Life can be unpredictable, and it's important to adjust your objectives if circumstances change.

Seek professional guidance: If needed, consult with a fitness professional or healthcare provider to ensure your goals are safe and tailored to your individual needs.

Stay consistent and persistent: Consistency is key to achieving any fitness goal. Stick to your Wall Pilates routine and stay committed even when progress seems slow.

Track and evaluate progress: Keep a record of your sessions, measurements, and achievements. Regularly assessing your progress helps you stay on track and provides a clear sense of accomplishment.

Setting achievable goals is a personal journey. It's about what's meaningful and realistic for you. By following these tips, you're laying a solid foundation for a successful and fulfilling Wall Pilates practice.

WALL SQUATS FOR LOWER BODY STRENGTH

Here's a simple Wall Pilates exercise to help you get started:

INSTRUCTIONS

- Stand with your back against a sturdy, flat wall.
- Place your feet about hip-width apart and a few inches away from the wall.
- Slowly slide your body down the wall, bending your knees, until your thighs are parallel to the ground. Your knees should be directly above your ankles.
- Hold this position for 15-30 seconds or as long as feels comfortable.
- Push through your heels to stand back up, straightening your legs.

TIPS

- Keep your back flat against the wall throughout the exercise.
- Engage your core muscles for stability.
- Focus on controlled movements, avoiding rapid or jerky motions.
- Breathe steadily and rhythmically.

This exercise targets the muscles in your legs, particularly the quadriceps, hamstrings, and glutes. It's an excellent starting point for building lower body strength, which is essential for stability and balance.

Remember; start with what feels comfortable for you and gradually increase the duration as you become more accustomed to the exercise. Always listen to your body and stop if you feel any discomfort or strain.

Now that you've grasped the fundamentals, it's time to dive in and start experiencing the benefits of Wall Pilates, beginning with an essential component: balance. This foundational aspect sets the stage for a solid and stable practice. Let's embark on this journey together, step by step, as we work toward a stronger, more flexible, and balanced you. Let's get started!

2

BALANCING ACTS

Phyllis's vintage personal trainer, Kristy, had this amazing story to share about her (Belanger, n.d.).

"Phyllis is a client who approaches her training with great intuition about her body, making our sessions both enjoyable and productive. Through regular communication, she keeps me informed about her physical sensations, allowing me to tailor our sessions accordingly. As we address her postural compensations, including mild scoliosis, Phyllis has made adjustments in her daily activities like gardening and cleaning, becoming more efficient with minimal discomfort. In the rare instances where she does experience aches, she now knows which stretches and exercises can help alleviate tension and build strength.

Phyllis's progress is remarkable; her measurements reveal improved symmetry, particularly in key areas like her head, shoulder blades, and hips. Her flexibility has surged to four times its original level, a major milestone she set for herself. Equally impressive is her threefold enhancement in balance, demonstrated by her ability to stand on one leg for over two minutes, significantly reducing her risk of falling.

One of Phyllis's initial goals was to enhance upper-body strength. Previously unable to perform a single push-up from the floor, she can now confidently complete 10. Her grip strength rivals that of someone half her age, a testament to her dedication. Phyllis has surpassed expectations in overhead lifts, comfortably managing 30 repetitions with five-pound weights. Notably, she can sustain a plank position for over two minutes, showcasing remarkable improvements in upper body, core, and postural stability.

Phyllis's journey also reflects positive changes in body composition. She's shed eight pounds, reducing her body fat percentage by five points. Moreover, her muscle mass percentage now exceeds recommended levels for her age and gender. Her success is a testament to her consistent commitment to the exercises and stretches I've prescribed. Phyllis has rightfully prioritized her health, and the dividends are evident. I'm excited to continue supporting Phyllis as she tackles her next set of goals."

Now, it's your turn. Imagine what you can achieve with wall Pilates. Phyllis's journey is a testament to the incredible potential within each of us. Your path to strength, flexibility, and balance starts here. Let's embark on this transformative journey together.

BALANCE-BUILDING BASICS: IMPORTANCE AND ASSESSMENTS

As we navigate the winding paths of life, it becomes abundantly clear that balance is far more than a mere physical attribute. It is the heartbeat of a life that resonates with vibrancy, activity, and the cherished gift of independence. This truth particularly shines as we gather the wisdom that naturally accompanies the passage of time.

Consider, for a moment, the profound impact of balance. It is the silent force that empowers us to seize life's small joys with grace and poise. It's the unspoken assurance that allows us to reach for that top shelf effortlessly, to wander through nature's beauty without trepidation, and even to engage in the spirited play of our beloved grandchildren. Without balance, these seemingly simple endeavors could easily transform into formidable challenges.

Yet balance's influence extends far beyond the physical realm. It infiltrates the very essence of our being, harmonizing our mental and emotional landscapes. When we stand on steady ground, our minds find equilibrium, enabling us to face life's inevitable twists and turns with fortitude and resilience.

As we do, it's crucial to recognize that balance exercises are not merely an option but a fundamental necessity. Let's explore why integrating these exercises into your routine is an investment in your overall well-being and quality of life.

Fall Prevention: Statistics vividly underscore the potential risks associated with falls, particularly as we advance in age

(Callicutt, 2020). However, the empowering truth is that many of these falls are preventable. Through targeted balance exercises, you fortify the very foundation that supports your mobility, reducing the likelihood of accidents.

Enhanced Mobility: Balance exercises foster a sense of stability and confidence in your movements. Imagine being able to navigate through daily activities with a newfound ease and grace. From reaching for items on a high shelf to strolling through a park, the benefits of enhanced mobility are immeasurable.

Independence: Maintaining balance directly impacts your ability to perform routine tasks independently. This self-reliance not only preserves your sense of agency but also nurtures a profound sense of empowerment.

Cognitive well-being: The mind-body connection is a powerful force. Engaging in balance exercises stimulates cognitive functions, enhancing your mental acuity and sharpness. This holistic approach to well-being ensures that you're nurturing both your physical and mental health.

Postural integrity: Proper posture is the mainstay of a healthy, pain-free existence. Balance exercises aid in aligning your body, reducing strain on muscles and joints. This, in turn, can alleviate discomfort and enhance your overall comfort in daily activities.

Confidence and peace of mind: There's a profound sense of assurance that comes with knowing you have the physical capability to navigate life's challenges. By dedicating time to balance exercises, you're not only investing in your physical health but also nurturing a deep-seated confidence in your own abilities.

Longevity and quality of life: A balanced body is a resilient body. By incorporating these exercises into your routine, you're proactively investing in your long-term health and vitality. This commitment to your well-being ensures that you're not just adding years to your life but enhancing the quality of those years.

Simple Balance Assessments You Can Do at Home

Before we dive into the transformative world of wall Pilates, let's take a moment to gauge where you are in terms of balance. These simple at-home tests will provide valuable insights into your current level of stability. Remember, this is a starting point, and as you progress through the chapters, you'll revisit these assessments to witness your remarkable improvement.

Single-leg Leg test

Find a stable surface and stand on one leg. Lift your other foot slightly off the ground, keeping your hands by your sides. Hold this position for as long as you can, ideally aiming for 30 seconds.

This test assesses your ability to maintain balance on one leg, a crucial skill for various daily activities.

Four-Stage Balance Test

- Stand with your feet close together, side by side.
- Place your hands on your hips or let them hang by your side.
- Hold this position for 10 seconds.
- Position the heel of one foot to touch the side of the big toe of the other foot.
- Hold this position for 10 seconds.
- Switch the position of your feet and hold for another 10 seconds.
- Place one foot directly in front of the other so that the heel of one foot is touching the toes of the other.
- Hold this position for 10 seconds.
- Switch the position of your feet and hold for another 10 seconds.
- Lift one foot off the ground, bending the knee at a 45-degree angle.
- Hold this position for as long as you can, ideally aiming for 30 seconds.
- Switch to the other leg and repeat.

Tandem Walk Test:

Create a clear path in your home. Walk along this path, placing one foot directly in front of the other, as if you're walking on a tightrope. Aim to maintain a straight line without stumbling.

This test focuses on the coordination and balance required for precise movements.

Modified Sit-to-Stand Test

Begin by sitting in a sturdy chair. Without using your hands for support, stand up and then sit back down. Repeat this action five times as quickly as possible.

This test evaluates your lower body strength, a crucial component of overall stability.

BALANCE EXERCISES

Now that we've delved into the significance of balance and assessed your current level, let's embark on a journey of practical exercises designed to enhance your stability. These exercises are carefully crafted to gradually strengthen your muscles and improve your sense of equilibrium.

Wall Stand

This exercise focuses on building strength in your calf muscles, a key component for maintaining balance.

INSTRUCTIONS

- Stand close to the wall and press both hands flat against it for support.
- Slowly lift your heels off the floor, rising onto your tiptoes, and then gently lower your heels back down.
- Aim for 8–10 lifts and increase gradually as you gain endurance.

Wall-Assisted Knee Lifts

This exercise aids in getting accustomed to balancing on one leg, a crucial skill for various daily activities.

INSTRUCTIONS

- Stand next to the wall and use one hand for support.
- Slowly lift one knee up toward your chest. Bring it up as far as feels comfortable for you. This movement engages your leg and core muscles.
- Lower your lifted knee back down gently. Keep the movement controlled and steady. This completes one repetition of the exercise.
- Begin with 8–10 repetitions on each leg.

Wall Slides

Wall slides target the leg muscles, fortifying them and providing essential support for improved balance.

INSTRUCTIONS

- Stand with your back against the wall, feet hip-width apart.
- Slowly slide down the wall until you're in a slight squat position, then gently slide back up.
- Achieve 8–10 repetitions and gradually increase as you gain more stability.

Wall-Assisted Leg Swings

This exercise is excellent for improving hip mobility and refining your sense of balance. It's a dynamic movement that engages various muscle groups.

INSTRUCTIONS

- Stand next to the wall with one hand on it for support.
- Swing one leg forward and backward in a controlled manner.
- Aim for 8–10 swings on each leg for the start.

Side Wall Press

This exercise targets arm strength and stability. It's a great way to engage your upper-body muscles while also practicing controlled movements.

INSTRUCTIONS

- Stand sideways to the wall. Position yourself close enough so you can easily touch the wall with one hand.
- Place one hand on the wall. This hand will be your support during the exercise.
- Gently lean into the wall. Apply a controlled, steady pressure against the wall using your hand.
- Push yourself back to your original standing position. This completes one repetition of the exercise.
- Aim for 8–10 repetitions.

Standing Pilates Legwork

This exercise not only challenges your balance but also targets the muscles in your legs and hips. It promotes strength and stability in your lower body.

INSTRUCTIONS

- Begin by standing upright with your feet hip-width apart. Ensure your posture is aligned and engage your core muscles for stability.
- Lift one leg to the side. Keep the leg straight and raise it to a comfortable height. This engages your leg muscles.
- Gently lower the leg back down to the starting position. Control the descent, focusing on the movement.
- Now, lift the opposite leg to the side. Again, keep it straight and raise it to a comfortable height.
- Gently lower the leg back down. Maintain control throughout the movement.
- Begin with 8–10 lifts on each leg.

ELEVATING YOUR BALANCE GAME

The basic balance exercises provided lay the groundwork. However, to truly advance your balance, it's crucial to delve into more challenging exercises. I highly recommend mastering the simpler ones before venturing into the more demanding ones.

Wall Push-Ups

This exercise builds arm strength, which is crucial for maintaining balance.

INSTRUCTIONS

- Stand at arm's length away from the wall.
- Place your hands flat on the wall at shoulder height.
- Bend your elbows and slowly move your chest toward the wall.
- Then, push yourself back to the starting position.
- Begin with 10–12 repetitions and increase gradually as you achieve more endurance.

Side Leg Lifts

This exercise targets the hip muscles and improves balance.

INSTRUCTION

- Stand with your side close to the wall and extend your arm for support.
- Lift the leg farthest from the wall as high as you can.
- Lower it back down in a controlled manner.
- Achieve 10–12 lifts on each leg, or until you cannot lift your leg anymore.

Wall Planks

Wall planks strengthen your core, an essential component for overall balance.

INSTRUCTIONS

- Place your hands on the wall at shoulder height.
- Walk your feet back until your body forms a slight angle with the wall.
- Hold this plank position for a few seconds (about 10 seconds), focusing on keeping your body straight.
- Repeat this exercise and aim for 10–12 repetitions.

Toe Taps

This exercise helps you get accustomed to balancing on one foot, improving stability.

INSTRUCTIONS

- Stand close to the wall for support.
- Lift one foot and tap the toes against the wall, then switch feet.
- Begin with 10–12 lifts on each foot.

Wall Sits

Wall sits strengthen your leg muscles, which are crucial for maintaining balance.

INSTRUCTIONS

- Stand with your back against the wall.
- Slide down into a seated position, bending your knees to a 90-degree angle, and hold for a few seconds.
- aim for 10–12 sits.

Remember to perform each exercise with control and focus on maintaining proper form. As you become more comfortable, you can gradually increase the duration or repetitions. These exercises will challenge your balance and help improve your overall stability.

MINDFUL BALANCE: MEDITATION TECHNIQUES

As we journey toward improved balance, it's crucial to recognize that this journey isn't solely physical. Mental focus and inner equilibrium play an equally vital role. By incorporating meditation practices, we can enhance our ability to center ourselves, fostering a deeper connection between mind and body.

Inner Balance Meditation

Begin by finding a quiet and comfortable space. Close your eyes if you feel comfortable doing so. Take a moment to ground yourself, focusing on your breath. Inhale deeply and exhale slowly, allowing any tension to dissipate. Set an intention for this practice; it could be finding harmony, peace, or stability within. Visualize a radiant light at your center, expanding with each breath. Feel this light radiate through your entire being, instilling a sense of inner balance.

Chakra Meditations

Chakras, energy centers within our body, play a significant role in our overall well-being. Engaging in specific chakra meditations can help restore and maintain balance in these energy centers. By focusing on each chakra, you can align your energy flow, contributing to a greater sense of equilibrium.

Mindful Awareness

Engage in mindfulness practices to heighten your awareness of the present moment. Whether it's mindful breathing, body scans, or observing your thoughts without judgment, these practices help cultivate a focused and centered mind.

By intertwining these meditation techniques with your physical balance exercises, you'll create a holistic approach to well-being. This synergy between mind and body will not only enhance your physical stability but also nurture a profound sense of inner harmony.

In this chapter, we've delved into the foundations of balance, understanding its pivotal role in leading an active and independent life, especially as we age. We've explored a range of exercises, from basic to more challenging, all designed to strengthen your stability and confidence. Additionally, we've introduced meditation techniques that not only enhance your physical balance but also foster a deeper connection between mind and body. As you progress on this journey, remember that achieving balance isn't just a physical feat; it's a mindful endeavor that encompasses your entire being.

Great balance is just the start. Next, let's straighten up with perfect posture in Wall Pilates. Get ready to discover how this foundational element sets the stage for a stronger, more confident you.

3

POSTURE PERFECT

Have you ever considered the profound impact good posture can have on your overall well-being? It's not just about standing up straight; it's about aligning your body in a way that supports your health and vitality.

Good posture is not a mere aesthetic concern; it's the anchor of a healthy, active life. When your body is properly aligned, you'll notice an increase in energy levels, a reduction in aches and pains, and a newfound sense of confidence. Whether you're a beginner or well-versed in Pilates, these exercises tailored for the wall will guide you toward achieving posture perfection.

Let me share a story that vividly illustrates the difference good posture can make in our daily lives. Meet Sue, a dedicated mother and professional who, like many of us, found herself battling with persistent back pain. It wasn't until she committed to improving her posture that she experienced a remarkable transformation. As her posture improved, so did her energy levels and overall sense of well-being. Through Wall Pilates, she discovered a holistic approach to not only alleviate her back pain but to enhance her quality of life.

UNDERSTANDING GOOD POSTURE: IMPACT AND ASSESSMENT

In our pursuit of a healthier, more vibrant life, few things are as fundamental as good posture. It's not just about appearances; it's about the very foundation upon which your health and well-being stand. Let's delve into what good posture truly entails and why it holds such paramount importance.

Good posture is more than simply standing up straight. It's about aligning your body in a way that maintains the natural curves of your spine, allowing for optimal function of your muscles, joints, and organs. When achieved, it fosters a state of equilibrium that positively influences your entire physical and mental well-being.

The benefits of good posture permeate every facet of our lives. When in proper alignment, the muscles and ligaments work harmoniously, distributing weight and pressure evenly. However, poor posture disrupts this balance, leading to overuse of certain muscles and strain on ligaments. Over time, this imbalance can result in chronic pain and discomfort, affecting your day-to-day activities. By cultivating good posture, you're essentially recalibrating your body's mechanics, allowing it to function optimally and without unnecessary strain.

Good posture plays a pivotal role in the efficient functioning of two essential bodily functions: Breathing and digestion. When you stand or sit upright, your lungs have ample space to expand and contract, ensuring a steady flow of oxygen to fuel your body. Additionally, proper alignment supports the natural position of your digestive organs, facilitating smooth digestion and absorption of nutrients. This means that good posture isn't just about appearances; it's about enhancing the very processes that sustain your life.

Consider the posture of someone you admire, be it a revered leader, a renowned athlete, or a beloved mentor. What do they have in common? They exude confidence and poise, standing tall and commanding attention. Good posture is an outward manifestation of inner strength and self-assuredness. When you carry yourself with an upright, aligned stance, you radiate an aura of confidence that is palpable to those around you. It's a silent but powerful declaration of your self-worth.

Self-Assessment: A Mirror to Your Posture

Posture, like many aspects of our physical well-being, can often be overlooked in the ebb and flow of daily life. Taking a moment to assess your own posture is a crucial step toward improvement.

Step 1: Select a quiet space where you have enough room to stand comfortably and where you can use a mirror. This will allow you to observe your posture from various angles.

Step 2: Begin by standing in your usual, relaxed posture. Let your arms hang naturally by your sides. Resist the urge to consciously adjust your stance at this point, as we want to capture your posture in its most natural state.

Step 3: Direct your attention to your shoulders. Are they slouched or rounded forward? Visualize an imaginary line across your shoulders; ideally, this line should be level and parallel to the ground. If you notice your shoulders hunching forward, this may be an indicator that your posture could benefit from some adjustments.

Step 4: Next, focus on your spine. Is it overly arched or hunched? A healthy spine maintains its natural curvature, forming a gentle "S" shape. If you observe an exaggerated arch or a pronounced rounding of your back, these may be signs that your posture could be improved.

Step 5: Pay attention to any discomfort or tension you might be feeling. This can be a valuable indicator of areas where your posture may be placing undue stress on your body.

Step 6: Mentally note your observations. This initial self-assessment serves as a baseline for your posture improvement journey.

Remember, this is not a judgment, but an opportunity for self-awareness. By recognizing areas that may need adjustment, you're taking an active step toward better posture and ultimately, improved well-being.

In the following sections of this chapter, we'll explore targeted Wall Pilates exercises designed to guide your body toward its natural, balanced state gently. Each exercise is tailored to address specific areas, ensuring a holistic approach to posture improvement.

IMPROVING POSTURE: WALL PILATES EXERCISES

Wall Angels

Let's begin with an exercise that not only engages your entire upper body but also promotes optimal shoulder alignment.

- Stand with your feet about hip-width apart, with your back against a flat wall.
- Ensure your head, shoulders, and hips are in contact with the wall.
- Extend your arms out to the sides, creating a "T" shape with your body.
- Bend your elbows at a 90-degree angle, bringing your hands toward the wall.
- Slowly slide your arms upward along the wall while maintaining the 90-degree angle at your elbows.
- Imagine you're making "snow angels" on the wall.
- Continue the movement until your arms are extended overhead, without allowing your back to arch away from the wall.
- Hold this position for a moment to feel the stretch in your shoulders.
- Slowly reverse the motion, bringing your arms back down to the starting position.

Key Tips

- Focus on keeping your entire back, especially your lower back, in contact with the wall throughout the movement.
- Engage your core muscles to prevent excessive arching of the lower back.
- Breathe steadily throughout the exercise, inhaling as you reach up, and exhaling as you return to the starting position.

Wall Push-Ups

In our quest to improve posture and build strength, Wall Push-Ups emerge as a valuable addition. This exercise targets your upper body, particularly the chest, shoulders, and arms, without straining your back.

- Stand facing a flat, sturdy wall, about arm's length away.
- Place your feet hip-width apart and ensure they're firmly grounded.
- Extend your arms forward and place your palms flat against the wall, about shoulder-width apart.
- Keep your wrists aligned with your shoulders.
- Maintain a straight line from your head to your heels. Engage your core muscles to support your spine.
- Slowly bend your elbows, lowering your body toward the wall.
- Keep your body in a straight line and aim to bring your chest as close to the wall as comfortable.

- Push through your palms to straighten your arms, returning to the starting position.

Key Tips

- Focus on controlled movements throughout the exercise, both on the descent and ascent.
- Keep your gaze forward and avoid arching or sagging your back.
- Breathe steadily, inhaling on the way down and exhaling as you push back up.

Chin Tucks

This simple yet effective movement, performed with your back against the wall, targets and strengthens the muscles of your neck.

- Begin by standing with your back against a flat wall, ensuring your head, shoulders, and hips are in contact with the wall.
- Keep your feet shoulder-width apart and ensure they're firmly grounded.
- Start with your head in a neutral position, looking straight ahead.
- Gently draw your chin in toward your neck without tilting your head up or down.
- Imagine you're trying to create a double chin but without straining or causing discomfort.

- Hold this position for a few seconds, feeling the engagement in the muscles at the front of your neck.
- Slowly release the chin tuck and return to the neutral head position.

Key Tips

- Maintain a relaxed, natural facial expression throughout the exercise.
- Avoid any excessive force or tension; the movement should be controlled and comfortable.
- Breathe steadily and naturally, without holding your breath.

Wall Planks

As we continue our journey toward improved posture and overall strength, let's introduce the Wall Planks exercise. This powerful movement, where you hold a plank position against the wall, serves to align the spine and fortify your core.

- Begin by standing facing the wall, approximately an arm's length away.
- Place your palms flat against the wall, about shoulder-width apart.
- Step your feet back, keeping them hip-width apart. Your body should be in a straight line from head to heels.
- Activate your abdominal muscles by drawing your navel toward your spine. This stabilizes your torso.

- Maintain this position, ensuring your body remains in a straight line. Avoid any sagging or arching of your back.
- Keep your gaze directed toward the wall.
- Focus on controlled breathing. Inhale deeply through your nose, allowing your chest and abdomen to rise. Exhale slowly through your mouth.
- Aim to hold the plank for as long as you can maintain proper form. Note the duration for future reference.
- Over time, work on increasing the duration of the plank as your core strength improves.

Key Tips

- Pay attention to your hand placement on the wall to ensure stability.
- Keep your shoulders away from your ears to avoid unnecessary tension.
- If you feel excessive strain or discomfort, gently come out of the plank position.

Wall Sits

Let's introduce the Wall Sits exercise. This powerful isometric movement, akin to sitting in an imaginary chair against the wall, serves to maintain a straight spine and fortify the muscles of your legs.

- Begin by standing with your back against a flat, sturdy wall.

- Slowly slide your back down the wall, bending your knees, until your thighs are parallel to the ground. Imagine you're sitting on an invisible chair.
- Ensure your knees are directly above your ankles, forming a 90-degree angle.
- Your feet should be hip-width apart and flat on the ground.
- Maintain a straight spine, avoiding any rounding or arching of your back. Your lower back should be in contact with the wall.
- Engage your leg muscles and hold this position for as long as you can maintain proper form.
- Keep your arms relaxed by your sides or on your thighs for support.
- Focus on controlled breathing. Inhale deeply through your nose, and exhale slowly through your mouth.
- Over time, work on increasing the duration of your wall sit as your leg strength improves.

Key Tips

- Keep your weight evenly distributed between both legs.
- Ensure your knees do not extend beyond your toes to protect your knee joints.
- If you experience discomfort or strain, gently stand up and take a short break.

CONFIDENCE AND POSTURE: SELF-CONFIDENCE BENEFITS

Have you ever considered the profound link between posture and self-confidence? It turns out that standing tall and maintaining good posture isn't just about appearances; it significantly impacts how we perceive ourselves and how others perceive us.

When we consciously choose to stand tall and maintain an upright posture, we set off a remarkable chain of physiological responses within our bodies. This response has been extensively studied and the findings are quite compelling.

Firstly, let's consider testosterone, a hormone often associated with vitality, assertiveness, and self-assuredness. When we stand upright, research has demonstrated a notable increase in testosterone levels. This surge in testosterone isn't merely coincidental; it's a direct result of our body's response to the powerful message conveyed by our posture.

On the flip side, there's cortisol, a hormone intricately linked with stress. When we maintain good posture, studies have shown a distinct decrease in cortisol levels. This reduction in cortisol is particularly significant, as it signifies a decrease in our body's stress response. This hormonal shift plays a pivotal role in fostering a profound sense of confidence and reducing feelings of anxiety and stress.

In essence, by standing tall and maintaining an upright posture, we're effectively orchestrating a hormonal symphony within ourselves. This shift in hormone levels not only empowers us with a sense of self-assurance but also affords us the physiological means to combat stress and anxiety (Ohio State University, 2009).

Proper posture not only affects testosterone and cortisol but also impacts other key hormones. For example, maintaining good posture can lead to an increase in dopamine, often referred to as the "feel-good" hormone. This surge in dopamine contributes to a more positive mood and greater self-assurance.

The profound connection between posture and cognitive function is a testament to the intricate interplay between our physical and mental well-being. Studies have consistently demonstrated that maintaining good posture is not only beneficial for our physical health but also holds remarkable implications for our cognitive abilities.

When we adopt an upright stance and consciously maintain good posture, we set in motion a series of cognitive advantages. Research suggests that this posture is associated with heightened brainpower. In essence, standing tall positively influences our cognitive performance, impacting various aspects of our mental abilities.

The benefits of this are far-reaching. Improved cognitive function is essential in navigating the complexities of our daily lives. It enhances our ability to process information, make decisions, and tackle challenges with clarity and efficiency. This, in turn, contributes to a heightened sense of confidence and assurance in various situations (Enterprise, 2014).

The way we carry ourselves in the world serves as a silent but powerful language. It communicates volumes about our confidence, self-assuredness, and readiness to engage with others. One of the remarkable aspects of good posture is how it influences the feedback we receive from the world around us.

When we stand tall and exude confidence through our posture, we send a clear signal to others. It's as if we're saying, "I am capable, self-assured, and ready to face whatever comes my way." This projection of confidence often leads to a distinct shift in the way others interact with us.

Consider this scenario: You walk into a room with your head held high, shoulders back, and a strong, purposeful stride. It's likely that you'll be met with warm smiles, open body language, and a positive, welcoming atmosphere. This is the immediate feedback you receive from your environment, and it's a direct response to the confidence you project through your posture.

Additionally, studies have shown that individuals with good posture are often perceived as more competent and capable by others. This perception can boost self-confidence, as it aligns with how we want to be perceived in both personal and professional settings (Enterprise, 2014).

Now that we've mastered the art of perfect posture, it's time to pivot toward another crucial element of overall well-being: Flexibility. In the upcoming chapters, we'll delve into how Wall Pilates can liberate our movements, allowing us to experience a newfound sense of freedom and suppleness. Let's embark on this journey toward enhanced flexibility and embrace the boundless potential it holds for our physical well-being.

4

FLEXIBILITY AND FREEDOM

I n this chapter, we embark on a journey to explore the crucial role that flexibility plays in our daily lives and overall health. You may wonder why flexibility matters and how it can contribute to your well-being.

Flexibility is not merely about contorting our bodies into pretzel-like shapes. It is about granting ourselves the freedom to move with ease, grace, and without constraint. Think about the simple act of reaching down to tie your shoelaces or turning to grab something from a high shelf. These seemingly mundane tasks become effortless and pain-free when you possess good flexibility.

Beyond these day-to-day activities, flexibility extends its benefits to our posture, balance, and even mental well-being. It allows us to adapt to life's challenges, both physically and mentally, with resilience and confidence.

Flexibility plays a pivotal role in achieving and maintaining proper posture. When muscles are flexible, they can move and adjust more freely, allowing you to comfortably hold your body in an upright position. This, in turn, reduces the likelihood of developing postural issues such as rounded shoulders or an arched back.

Flexibility is closely intertwined with balance. Imagine a tight, inflexible muscle trying to support you in a challenging balance pose; it's like trying to balance on a rigid pillar. However, when your muscles are pliable and adaptable, they can respond more effectively to shifts in weight and movement, providing you with greater stability.

Furthermore, improved flexibility is not just a physical achievement, but a profound investment in your health. It enhances blood circulation, reduces the risk of injuries, and alleviates muscle tension. Moreover, it promotes better joint health and posture, which can have a positive ripple effect on your overall sense of well-being.

Life is an ever-changing journey, filled with unexpected twists and turns. Flexibility in both body and mind equips you to navigate these changes with greater ease. Whether it's a sudden change in routine, a physical demand, or a mental hurdle, your flexibility allows you to adjust and respond in a way that minimizes stress and strain. It's the difference between being a rigid tree that may break in a storm and a supple reed that can bend and sway, emerging stronger after the tempest.

FLEXIBILITY BASICS: GETTING STARTED

Flexibility refers to the ability of our muscles and joints to move through their full range of motion. It's about the suppleness and adaptability of our bodies, allowing us to perform a wide array of movements with ease and without strain. Picture the effortless reach for an object on a high shelf, the graceful bend to tie your shoes, or the smooth, unhindered motion of walking. All of these actions are made possible by flexibility.

Flexibility is not a luxury reserved for athletes or dancers; it is a fundamental aspect of physical health and well-being for everyone, at every stage of life. Improved flexibility allows you to move your limbs and joints freely in all directions. This means you can engage in a broader range of activities, from simple daily tasks to more dynamic physical pursuits.

When your muscles and joints are flexible, they are less likely to become strained or injured during physical activity. This is because they can adapt to sudden movements or changes in direction, preventing undue stress on tissues.

Understanding Range of Motion: Vital for Seniors

Range of motion (ROM) refers to the extent to which a joint or a group of joints can move in various directions. It encompasses the flexion, extension, rotation, and other movements that our bodies are capable of. For instance, the ability to raise your arm overhead, bend your knees, or rotate your neck are all examples of different ranges of motion.

Maintaining an optimal range of motion becomes increasingly vital as we age, and here is why:

Preservation of independence: A healthy range of motion is directly linked to your ability to perform daily activities independently. Tasks like dressing, bathing, reaching for objects, and even getting in and out of chairs rely on your joints' ability to move freely.

Prevention of joint stiffness: Without regular movement, joints tend to become stiff and less pliable. This stiffness can lead to discomfort, pain, and a decreased ability to move comfortably.

Reduced risk of falls: Adequate range of motion is a key component of balance and stability. This means that having a full range of motion can significantly reduce the risk of falls and accidents, which can have serious consequences for seniors.

Alleviation of pain and discomfort: Limited range of motion often leads to muscle imbalances and increased joint stress. This can result in chronic pain and discomfort, which can be particularly challenging for seniors.

Improved circulation: Full movement of joints helps maintain healthy blood flow, ensuring that nutrients and oxygen reach your muscles and tissues efficiently.

Enhanced quality of Life: Being able to move freely and comfortably significantly contributes to your overall well-being and enjoyment of life. It allows you to engage in activities that bring you joy and fulfillment.

Assessing Your Flexibility: Where You Stand

Before we embark on your journey toward improved flexibility through Wall Pilates, it's crucial to take a moment to assess your current level of flexibility. This will serve as a starting point and a valuable reference as you progress on this transformative path.

Shoulder Mobility Test

- Stand with your feet shoulder-width apart.
- Raise one arm straight up overhead.
- Bend your elbow and reach your hand down your back.
- With the other hand, try to reach up your back and touch your fingertips together.
- Note how far apart your hands are. Repeat on the other side.

This test assesses the flexibility of your shoulders and upper back.

Toe Touch Test

- Stand with your feet together and legs straight.
- Slowly bend forward at your waist and try to touch your toes.
- Take note of how far you can comfortably reach.

This test evaluates the flexibility of your hamstrings and lower back.

Hip Flexor Stretch

- Kneel on one knee with the other foot in front, forming a 90-degree angle.
- Gently push your hips forward until you feel a stretch in the front of your hip on the kneeling leg.
- Hold for 15-30 seconds and switch legs.

This stretch targets the hip flexors, which can often be tight.

Seated Forward Bend

- Sit with your legs extended straight in front of you.
- Slowly bend forward at your hips, reaching toward your toes.
- Note how far you can comfortably reach.

This stretch helps assess hamstring and lower back flexibility.

These assessments offer valuable insights into your current level of flexibility. They can help identify areas that may benefit from targeted Wall Pilates exercises. Remember, flexibility varies from person to person, and there is no right or wrong level. The aim is to improve and enhance your own range of motion gradually.

FLEXIBILITY EXERCISES: SIMPLE STRETCHES

Now that we've laid the groundwork, it's time to dive into some beginner-friendly Wall Pilates exercises that are specifically tailored to enhance your flexibility. These stretches are gentle, effective, and perfect for those who are just starting their journey.

Wall Calf Stretch

This stretch targets the calf muscles, which can become tight due to various activities and lack of regular stretching.

- Stand facing a wall, keeping a comfortable distance.
- Place your hands against the wall at shoulder height. This provides support and stability during the stretch.
- Take one foot and step it back a comfortable distance. Ensure both feet are flat on the ground.
- Press the heel of your back foot into the floor. This helps to engage the calf muscles.
- Keep your back leg straight while slightly bending the front knee.
- You should feel a gentle, elongating stretch in the calf of your back leg. It's important not to push too hard; a mild stretch is sufficient.
- Hold this position for about 15-30 seconds while taking slow, deep breaths.
- Release the stretch, step your other foot back, and repeat the process on the opposite side.

Remember, the key is to go at your own pace and never force a stretch. It's perfectly normal if you can't go as far as you'd like initially. With consistent practice, you'll notice an improvement in your flexibility.

Wall Hamstring Stretch

This stretch is particularly beneficial for increasing the suppleness of the back of your thigh and lower back.

- Sit on the floor with one leg extended straight out in front of you and the other bent, sole against the wall.
- The sole of your bent leg should rest comfortably against the wall. This provides support and stability during the stretch.
- Keeping your back straight, gently reach toward the toe of your extended leg.
- As you reach, you should feel a gentle yet effective stretch along the back of your thigh and possibly into your lower back.
- Hold this position for about 15-30 seconds. It's important to find a point of stretch that feels comfortable and sustainable. Avoid pushing yourself too hard.
- Release the stretch, switch the position of your legs, and repeat the process on the opposite side.

As you engage in this stretch, take a moment to breathe deeply and let go of any tension. Allow yourself to sink into the stretch, and with each breath, feel the release and increased flexibility.

Wall Shoulder Opener

This stretch is designed to release tension across your chest and shoulders. Follow these steps:

- Stand with your side facing the wall.
- Extend your arm and place your hand flat against the wall.
- Turn your body gently away from the wall. You should feel a stretch across your chest and shoulder.
- Maintain this position for about 15-30 seconds, taking slow, deep breaths.

Wall-Assisted Quad Stretch

This stretch targets the front of your thigh, an area often tight for many individuals. Here's how you do it:

- Stand facing away from the wall.
- Bend one knee and bring the foot up toward your glutes.
- Use the wall for balance as you hold the ankle with your hand. Ensure your knees are close together.
- You should feel a stretch along the front of your thigh.
- Maintain this position for about 15-30 seconds, allowing the stretch to deepen with each breath.

Wall Inner Thigh Stretch

- Sit down with your back against the wall.
- Place the soles of your feet together, letting your knees drop out to the sides.
- Use your hands to press down gently on your knees.

These stretches are wonderful additions to your flexibility routine. Remember, consistency is key. As you practice, you'll notice an improvement in your range of motion and a newfound sense of ease in your movements.

ADVANCING FLEXIBILITY: THE NEXT LEVEL

As you continue on your journey toward enhanced flexibility, it's time to introduce some more advanced Wall Pilates exercises. These exercises are designed to challenge and further expand your range of motion, ultimately leading to increased stretch and agility.

Wall Lunge Stretch

The Wall Lunge Stretch is a dynamic exercise that focuses on your lower body, particularly your hips and thighs.

- Stand a few feet away from a wall.
- Take one foot and step it forward into a lunge position. Ensure your knee is directly above your ankle.
- Place your hands on the wall above your head. This provides support and helps maintain balance.

- Gently lean your body toward the wall. This will deepen the stretch, particularly in your hip flexors and thigh muscles.
- You should feel a strong yet comfortable stretch in the front of your hip and thigh of the extended leg.
- Hold this position for about 15-30 seconds, breathing deeply to allow the stretch to settle.

Extended Wall Calf Stretch

This variation takes the familiar Wall Calf Stretch to a new level, providing a more intense stretch for your calf muscles.

- Stand facing a wall, maintaining a comfortable distance.
- Begin by following the steps for the basic Wall Calf Stretch: Place your hands against the wall, step one foot back, and press the heel into the floor. Keep the back leg straight and bend the front knee slightly until you feel a stretch in the calf of the back leg.
- Now, to take it to the next level, lift the ball of your back foot off the ground. This action intensifies the stretch in your calf.
- As you lift the ball of your foot, focus on maintaining your balance and control. Use the wall for support if needed.
- You should feel a more pronounced and concentrated stretch in your calf muscles.
- Hold this position for about 15-30 seconds, breathing deeply to allow the stretch to settle.

Wall Splits

This stretch offers a unique opportunity to challenge your flexibility and reach for greater heights in your range of motion.

- Begin by standing with your side facing the wall.
- Extend one leg up the wall while keeping the other leg straight on the ground. Your body will form an 'L' shape.
- Gently lean into the stretch, aiming to get your chest as close to the wall as possible. This action deepens the stretch and intensifies the sensation.
- Only go as far as your body allows. You should feel a stretch along the back of your extended leg, particularly in your hamstrings.
- Take slow, deep breaths and hold this position for about 15-30 seconds.

Wall Hip Opener

This stretch targets your hip flexibility, a crucial aspect of overall mobility. Let's walk through the steps together.

- Stand facing the wall with your hands against it. Maintain a comfortable distance.
- Begin by lifting one knee toward your chest. Keep your core engaged for stability.
- From this raised position, gently open your knee out to the side. This motion should be controlled and deliberate.

- Focus on keeping your hips square, meaning they should be parallel to the wall. This ensures you're targeting the hip flexors effectively.
- You should feel a deep stretch in the hip of the raised leg and possibly into the inner thigh as well.
- Maintain this position for about 15-30 seconds, taking slow, deep breaths.

Wall Cobra Stretch

This exercise invites you to open up your heart, stretch your abdominal muscles, and promote a sense of vitality.

- Begin by lying face down on the floor with your hands positioned against the bottom of the wall.
- Your hands should be slightly wider than shoulder-width apart, with your palms flat against the wall.
- Engage your arms and press up, as if you were doing a push-up. However, keep your hips firmly on the floor.
- As you press up, allow your chest to open and lift toward the wall. This action stretches your abdominal muscles.
- Be mindful to keep your hips grounded. The stretch should primarily be felt in your abdominal region.
- Hold this position for about 15-30 seconds, taking slow, deep breaths.

The Wall Cobra is a powerful exercise that not only promotes flexibility but also encourages a sense of openness and vitality.

As you perform this stretch, visualize your heart center expanding, inviting in a renewed sense of energy.

MINDFUL FLEXIBILITY: CALM YOUR MIND, STRETCH YOUR BODY

As we progress on this journey of flexibility and well-being, it's essential to introduce the concept of mindful stretching. This approach involves more than just the physical act of stretching; it invites you to engage your mind in the process, creating a harmonious connection between body and spirit.

Mindful stretching entails being fully present in each movement, paying keen attention to the sensations in your body, and cultivating a sense of inner calm.

By tuning into the sensations during a stretch, you become more attuned to the subtle nuances of your body's movements. This heightened awareness allows for a deeper and more effective stretch.

When you approach stretching with mindfulness, you're less likely to rush through it. This allows for a more gradual and sustained release of tension, ultimately leading to improved flexibility.

Additionally, engaging in mindful stretching shifts your focus away from worries and stressors, providing a mental respite. The rhythmic flow of breath and movement induces a state of calm and relaxation.

Moreover, mindful stretching deepens the connection between your physical body and your mind. This synergy fosters a sense of unity and balance, promoting overall well-being.

Cultivating Calmness: Relaxation Techniques in Wall Pilates

In our journey toward enhanced flexibility and well-being, it's vital to incorporate relaxation techniques that complement your Wall Pilates practice. These techniques will not only deepen the benefits of your stretches but also offer a profound sense of calmness and tranquility. Let's explore some simple yet effective ways to integrate relaxation into your routine.

Deep Breathing

As you move through your Wall Pilates stretches, focus on your breath. Inhale deeply through your nose, allowing your abdomen to rise, and exhale slowly through your mouth, releasing any tension. This rhythmic breathing pattern calms the nervous system, promoting relaxation.

Mindful Visualization

During each stretch, visualize the targeted muscles lengthening and relaxing. Imagine them becoming more flexible and supple with each breath. This mental imagery enhances the mind-body connection and encourages a deeper release of tension.

Progressive Muscle Relaxation

As you hold a stretch, consciously relax the muscles not involved in the stretch. Start from your toes and work your way up to your head, releasing any unnecessary tension. This technique encourages a profound sense of relaxation throughout your body.

Guided Meditation

Consider incorporating short, guided meditation sessions into your practice. Before or after your Wall Pilates routine, take a few minutes to sit in a quiet space and listen to a guided meditation focused on relaxation and mindfulness.

Affirmations

Pair positive affirmations with your stretches. As you hold a stretch, repeat affirming statements to yourself, such as "I am calm and at ease," or "My body is becoming more flexible with each breath." This reinforces a positive mindset and encourages relaxation.

Improving your flexibility is a significant achievement, and as you've discovered, the power of relaxation and mindfulness plays a crucial role. However, there's another tool that's just as vital: Your breath. In the next chapter, we'll delve deeper into the art of breath control and how mastering it can take your Wall Pilates practice and overall well-being to even greater heights.

As you conclude this chapter, take a moment to appreciate the progress you've made in enhancing your flexibility. These exercises are the pathway to newfound freedom in your movements.

Consistency is your ally. The more you integrate these practices into your daily routine, the more profound the effects will become. Each stretch and extension nurtures your body toward a state of increased flexibility and vitality.

Remember, this journey doesn't end here. While flexibility is a significant milestone, there's another crucial tool at your disposal: Your breath. In the next chapter, we'll delve into how mastering breath control can further elevate your Wall Pilates practice and enhance your overall well-being.

5

BREATH CONTROL

Take a deep breath. Feel the air fill your lungs, expanding your chest and releasing any tension. This simple act holds immense power, not only for your Wall Pilates practice but for your overall well-being.

Imagine a scenario: Think of two individuals, one breathing shallowly and the other with purposeful, deep breaths. The first struggles through their exercises, muscles tense and movements restricted. The second moves gracefully, each motion harmonizing with their breath, creating a seamless flow of energy and control.

In this chapter, we embark on a journey into the realm of controlled breathing, the foundation of Wall Pilates. Controlled breathing, as you'll discover, is not confined to the realm of Wall Pilates. It permeates every facet of your existence. It is the anchor that steadies you in moments of chaos, the balm that soothes your mind, and the fuel that ignites your inner strength.

Through controlled breathing, you gain agency over your responses. You navigate challenges with poise and respond to life's ebbs and flows with grace. It's a tool that empowers you to find calm amidst the storm and cultivate clarity in moments of confusion.

On a physical level, controlled breathing optimizes the flow of oxygen to your muscles, invigorating them with each inhale. It allows for smoother, more efficient movement in your Pilates practice, unlocking new levels of strength and flexibility.

But it doesn't stop there. Your breath is a gateway to your emotional landscape. It is intimately connected to your stress response, influencing your heart rate, blood pressure, and overall sense of well-being. With conscious breath, you hold the reins to your emotional state, enabling you to navigate through challenges with composure.

In moments of stillness, your breath becomes a source of intro-spection, a guide to the depths of your inner world. It invites you to connect with your true self, offering clarity and insight.

Our breath is more than an automatic function; it's a powerful tool we can harness to improve our health and enrich our lives. As we explore various breathing techniques, you'll uncover how this fundamental practice can transform your Pilates journey and leave a positive imprint on your day-to-day life.

PROGRESSIVE EXERCISES: BASIC TO ADVANCED BREATHING

Now that we've uncovered the transformative power of controlled breathing, it's time to put it into action with a series of progressive exercises. These exercises will take you from basic techniques to more advanced practices, allowing you to gradually deepen your breath control and enhance your Wall Pilates experience.

Complete Breathing

This foundational exercise lays the groundwork for controlled breathing.

- Find a quiet space where you can sit or stand comfortably.
- Inhale deeply through your nose, allowing your abdomen to expand as your lungs fill with air.
- Exhale slowly through slightly pursed lips, ensuring a gentle release of the breath.

Humming Breathing

This exercise introduces a controlled vocal element to your breath, enhancing its depth and resonance.

- Begin by finding a comfortable position that allows you to be at ease.

- Take a moment to inhale deeply, allowing your lungs to fill with refreshing air.
- As you exhale, produce a gentle humming sound. Feel the vibrations resonate within you.

This exercise not only enriches your breath but also invites a sense of focused tranquility.

Purse-Lipped Breathing

This technique refines control over the exhale, promoting relaxation and focus.

- Adopt a comfortable stance, ensuring your body is at ease.
- Inhale through your nose, then exhale gently through pursed lips, as if blowing out a candle.

Balanced Breathing

This exercise emphasizes symmetrical inhalation and exhalation, promoting a sense of equilibrium.

- Stand or sit with feet firmly rooted.
- Inhale for a count of four, allowing your breath to fill both sides of your body equally.
- Exhale with the same deliberate rhythm, maintaining a sense of balance throughout.

Feet Breathing

This advanced exercise combines breath awareness with focused imagery, creating a deeply grounding experience.

- Find a quiet space and take a moment to center yourself.
- Close your eyes and envision your breath flowing down to your feet as you inhale, then back up as you exhale.

Remember, progression is a personal journey. Listen to your body and adjust the exercises to suit your comfort level. With dedication, these breathing techniques will become second nature, enriching your Wall Pilates practice and enhancing your overall well-being.

Tips on How to Sync These Breathing Exercises With Wall Pilates Moves

Now that you're acquainted with these powerful breathing exercises, let's explore how to integrate them into your Wall Pilates routine seamlessly. This synchronization not only enhances the effectiveness of your practice but also fosters a deeper mind-body connection.

Mindful preparation: Before you begin any Pilates move, take a moment to center yourself. Stand or sit in your chosen position and initiate a few rounds of Complete Breathing. This sets the stage for a focused and intentional practice.

Rhythmic harmony: As you transition into your Pilates movements, synchronize your breath with each motion. For instance, during an inhale, engage in a movement that expands or opens your body, and during an exhale, engage in a movement that contracts or draws your body inward. This rhythmic flow ensures that your breath supports and guides each action.

Match breath phases: Tailor your breathing to complement specific phases of a Pilates move. For example, during a challenging exertion phase, exhale to enhance your stability and control. Conversely, during a relaxation phase, inhale deeply to rejuvenate and prepare for the next movement.

Use sound as a guide: In exercises like Humming Breathing, allow the sound of your breath to serve as a rhythmical guide. The vibrations created by the hum can further enhance your awareness of breath flow, promoting a seamless integration with your Pilates routine.

Maintain a consistent pace: Ensure that your breath flows steadily and consistently throughout each movement. Avoid holding your breath, as this can lead to tension and disrupt the fluidity of your practice.

Listen to your body: Pay close attention to how your body responds to each breath. Adjust the pace and depth of your breath to match the intensity of the movement. This intuitive approach allows you to optimize your breath's support for your Pilates practice.

Keep in mind that the integration of breath and movement in Wall Pilates is a dynamic and personal practice. It enhances not only the physical benefits but also deepens your mental focus and presence.

REDUCING STRESS AND ENHANCING EMOTIONAL HEALTH

Your breath is a multifaceted tool, serving as a bridge between your physical and emotional realms. When approached with intention, it carries the potential to harmonize these aspects of your being.

In moments of turbulence, whether physical discomfort or emotional unrest, your breath offers a sanctuary. Deep, controlled inhalations and exhalations send a powerful signal to your nervous system. They convey a message of assurance, a proclamation that all is well in this moment. In response, your body eases its production of stress hormones, creating a profound shift toward calmness.

Imagine it as a gentle hand on your shoulder, assuring you that you are safe, grounded, and capable of weathering any storm. In this way, your breath serves as a steadfast anchor, allowing you to find solace amidst life's challenges.

The rhythmic dance of inhalations and exhalations acts as a tether, drawing you into the present moment. In this sacred space, worries about the past lose their grip, and anxieties about the future dissipate. All that remains is the here and now, where life unfolds.

Within this present moment, you gain access to a heightened awareness of your emotions. You become attuned to their ebbs and flows, recognizing them as passing visitors rather than defining characteristics. This mindful presence grants you a precious pause, a moment of clarity in which you can choose how to respond to the circumstances at hand.

With this heightened awareness, you step into a realm of empowered choice. Instead of reacting impulsively to challenges or emotions, you have the space to respond thoughtfully. You hold the reins of your own narrative, making decisions from a place of centeredness and wisdom.

In this way, your breath becomes a conduit for mindful living. It guides you to navigate life's intricacies with grace and presence, allowing you to engage in a way that aligns with your truest self.

A Mindfulness Exercise: The Three-Minute Breathing Space

Here's a simple yet impactful exercise to integrate into your daily routine:

Grounding (1 minute): Begin by taking a moment to ground yourself. Close your eyes and take a deep breath in, allowing your awareness to settle into your body. Feel the contact of your feet with the ground, your hands resting on your lap, and the gentle rise and fall of your chest with each breath.

Observing (1 minute): Shift your attention to your breath. Notice the natural rhythm of your inhales and exhales. Pay close attention to the sensation of the breath entering and leaving your body. Let go of any judgments or attempts to change your breath; simply observe.

Expanding awareness (1 minute): Gradually expand your awareness to your surroundings. Notice the sounds around you, the sensations in your body, and any emotions that may be present. Allow everything to coexist without attachment or resistance.

This exercise serves as a powerful reset button, allowing you to step back from the rush of daily life and reconnect with your inner calm.

HOW BREATH CONTROL WORKS

At its core, breath control hinges on a delicate interplay between your respiratory system, nervous system, and musculature. When you take a conscious breath, you engage your diaphragm—a dome-shaped muscle beneath your ribcage. As you inhale, your diaphragm contracts, expanding the thoracic cavity and drawing air into your lungs. When you exhale, the diaphragm relaxes, allowing air to be expelled.

This intentional control of breath influences your autonomic nervous system. Deep, controlled breaths activate the parasympathetic nervous system, often referred to as the "rest and digest" system. This response counters the sympathetic nervous system's "fight or flight" mode, reducing stress hormone production and inducing a sense of calm.

During exercise, controlled breathing is akin to a symphony conductor guiding your body's movements. By synchronizing breath with exertion, you optimize oxygen intake and carbon dioxide expulsion. This ensures your muscles receive the necessary oxygen to perform optimally and efficiently expel waste products.

Controlled breathing also stabilizes your core, enhancing posture and balance. It supports your body's structural integrity, allowing for controlled and precise movements.

Beyond exercise, intentional breath control has far-reaching benefits for your general well-being. It acts as a potent stress-reduction tool, moderating the body's response to perceived threats. This, in turn, lowers heart rate, blood pressure, and cortisol levels, contributing to a calmer state of being.

Moreover, controlled breathing fosters mental clarity and emotional balance. It cultivates a sense of mindfulness, enabling you to respond thoughtfully rather than react impulsively to life's challenges. This centered approach to living bolsters your emotional resilience and enhances your capacity for presence and joy.

NUTRITION TIPS

Optimal lung function is a cornerstone of overall well-being, and your choice of foods and drinks can play a crucial role in supporting this vital aspect of your health. Here are some nutrition tips to enhance lung function and make breathing feel easier:

Berries: Blueberries, strawberries, and raspberries are packed with antioxidants that can help reduce inflammation in the lungs and improve respiratory function.

Nuts and seeds: Almonds, walnuts, flaxseeds, and chia seeds are excellent sources of magnesium and antioxidants. They can help relax the muscles around the airways, making it easier to breathe.

Oranges and citrus fruits: These fruits are rich in vitamin C, which is known for its immune-boosting properties and can help protect the lungs from damage.

Ginger and turmeric: These spices have anti-inflammatory properties that can help reduce inflammation in the airways, potentially improving lung function.

Green tea: This antioxidant-rich beverage contains compounds that may help improve lung function and protect against respiratory infections.

Water: Staying well-hydrated is crucial for maintaining healthy lung function. Water helps keep the mucous membranes in your respiratory tract moist, making it easier to breathe.

Garlic: This aromatic herb contains allicin, a natural compound associated with anti-inflammatory and antioxidant effects, potentially benefiting lung health.

Avocado: Rich in potassium and magnesium, avocados can help relax the muscles around the airways, making breathing easier.

You've now equipped yourself with the knowledge to support your lung health through nutrition and breathing exercises. By incorporating these breathing techniques, foods and drinks into your diet, you're taking a significant step toward optimizing your respiratory function.

Remember, your lungs are a vital aspect of your overall well-being and nourishing them with the right exercises and nutrients can make a tangible difference.

As we move forward, it's time to transition our focus. You've mastered the art of breathing; let's use that good oxygen to build some muscle in the next chapter.

HOME-BASED WALL PILATES FOR BEGINNERS, SENIORS

EXERCISES TO INCREASE BALANCE, IMPROVE POSTURE, FLEXIBILITY, AND REINFORCE STABILITY FOR VISIBLE BODY TRANSFORMATION IN AS LITTLE AS 29-DAYS

"People who give without expectation live longer, happier lives and make more money. So if we've got a shot at that during our time together, darn it, I'm gonna try."

To make that happen, I have a question for you...

Would you help someone you've never met, even if you never got credit for it?

Who is this person you ask? They are like you. Or, at least, like you used to be. Less experienced, wanting to make a difference, and needing help, but not sure where to look.

Our mission is to make Home-Based Wall Pilates for Beginners, Seniors accessible to everyone. Everything we do stems from that mission. And, the only way for us to accomplish that mission is by reaching...well...everyone.

This is where you come in. Most people do, in fact, judge a book by its cover (and its reviews). So here's my ask on behalf of a struggling beginner or senior looking to enhance their well-being:

Please help that reader by leaving this book a review.

Your gift costs no money and less than 60 seconds to make real, but can change a fellow reader's life forever. Your review could help…

- … one more small business provide for their community.
- … one more entrepreneur support their family.
- … one more employee get meaningful work.
- … one more client transform their life.
- … one more dream come true.

To get that 'feel good' feeling and help this person for real, all you have to do is…and it takes less than 60 seconds… leave a review.

If you feel good about helping a faceless reader, you are my kind of person. Welcome to the club. You're one of us.

I'm that much more excited to help you improve your balance, posture, flexibility, and stability faster and easier than you can possibly imagine. You'll love the exercises and techniques I'm about to share in the coming chapters.

Thank you from the bottom of my heart. Now, back to our regularly scheduled programming.

Your biggest fan, Sebastian Castellanos

PS - Fun fact: If you provide something of value to another person, it makes you more valuable to them. If you'd like good-will straight from another reader - and you believe this book will help them - send this book their way

Scan the QR code below to leave your review!

6

STRENGTH TRAINING

S trength training is the rock of a vibrant, functional life, particularly in the context of Wall Pilates. It forms the backbone of your physical vitality, empowering you to perform daily tasks with ease and confidence. As we age, maintaining muscle mass and strength becomes paramount, and Wall Pilates offers a safe and effective platform to achieve this.

Meet Jake, a spirited 60-year-old whose life took an extraordinary turn when he embraced strength training through Wall Pilates. Initially, he approached it with a mix of curiosity and determination, unsure of what to expect.

As the weeks went by, something remarkable unfolded. Jake's days, once filled with moments of physical strain, started to feel more manageable. Tasks like lifting groceries or even getting in and out of his car became noticeably easier. It was as if a newfound vitality coursed through his veins.

But the changes weren't just physical. Jake's posture underwent a transformation, standing tall and proud, a testament to the strength building within. He moved through life with a grace and stability that seemed to defy the passage of time.

What was even more striking was the impact on Jake's mental well-being. There was a newfound confidence that radiated from him, an assurance that he could face whatever challenges life presented. He felt a vitality within him that transcended the physical; it was a deep-seated sense of aliveness that permeated every aspect of his being.

Strength training had become a pillar of Jake's life, a practice that not only revitalized his body but also revitalized his spirit. It was a reminder that age was not a limitation but rather an invitation to tap into reservoirs of potential waiting to be unleashed.

Jake's journey serves as a compelling testament to the transformative power of strength training, particularly within the realm of Wall Pilates. It's a reminder that, with commitment, the human body and spirit have an incredible capacity for rejuvenation.

As you embark on this chapter, remember that strength training is not about attaining the physique of a bodybuilder but rather about empowering yourself to live life to the fullest. It's about nurturing your body, safeguarding your independence, and fortifying your mental resilience.

Throughout this chapter, you will be introduced to a range of wall resistance exercises, starting from the basics and gradually progressing to more advanced techniques. These exercises are tailored to suit your unique needs, ensuring a safe and effective approach to building strength.

PROGRESSIVE EXERCISES: BUILDING STRENGTH STEP-BY-STEP

These exercises are tailored to suit individuals at every level, from beginners taking their first steps toward strength training to advanced practitioners seeking to further refine their prowess.

BEGINNER LEVEL

Exercise 1: Wall Push-Ups

- Stand facing the wall, arms extended at chest height.
- Step back a bit to create an angle.
- Inhale as you bend your elbows and lower your chest toward the wall.
- Exhale as you push yourself back to the starting position.

Exercise 2: Wall Leg Raises

- Stand facing the wall, maintaining a comfortable distance for balance.
- To make it easier, lightly rest your fingertips on the wall for balance and stability.
- Lift your right leg a few inches off the ground.

- Gently tap your toes against the wall.
- Slowly lower your right leg back down to the ground.
- Lift your left leg a few inches off the ground.
- Gently tap your toes against the wall.
- Slowly lower your left leg back down to the ground.
- Focus on controlled motions throughout the exercise to maintain balance and stability.
- Start with a lower number of repetitions, and gradually increase as you gain confidence and strength.

Exercise 3: Wall Standing Rows

- Stand facing the wall with your arms extended at shoulder height.
- Grip the wall with your hands and pull your body toward the wall.
- Slowly release yourself back to the starting position.

INTERMEDIATE LEVEL

Exercise 1: Wall Squat

- Stand with your back against the wall, feet shoulder-width apart.
- Slide down the wall, bending your knees until they're at a 90-degree angle.
- Hold this position for a few breaths.
- Inhale as you push through your heels to stand back up.

Exercise 2: Wall Sit with Leg Lifts

- Stand with your back against the wall, feet shoulder-width apart.
- Slide down into a wall sit position, with your knees bent at a 90-degree angle.
- Lift your right leg, straightening it out in front of you.
- Lower it back down and repeat with your left leg.

Exercise 3: Wall Push-Ups with Leg Raise

- Stand facing the wall, arms extended at chest height.
- Step back slightly to create an angle.
- Perform a push-up by bending your elbows and leaning toward the wall.
- As you push back, lift your right leg off the ground.
- Lower your leg and repeat the push-up, this time lifting your left leg.

These intermediate-level exercises add an extra challenge to your wall resistance training routine. Focus on maintaining proper form and controlled movements for maximum effectiveness.

ADVANCED LEVEL

Exercise 1: Wall Planks

- Assume a plank position with your forearms against the wall.
- Keep your body in a straight line from head to heels.
- Engage your core and hold this position for as long as you can.

Each of these exercises can be adapted to your current level of strength. Progress at your own pace, and don't hesitate to modify the exercises to suit your needs.

Exercise 2: Wall Handstand Push-Ups

- Begin in a handstand position with your feet against the wall and your hands on the ground.
- Slowly lower your head toward the ground, then push back up to the starting position.

Exercise 3: Wall Pike Press

- Start in a plank position with your feet against the wall and your hands on the ground, forming an inverted "V" shape.
- Lower the top of your head toward the ground, then push back up to the starting position.

These advanced-level exercises require a high level of strength, stability, and control. Make sure to practice them in a safe environment, and if needed, have a spotter or instructor assist you.

Tips for Form and Safety to Avoid Injury

Ensuring proper form and safety during your Wall Pilates practice is paramount to a successful and injury-free experience. Here are some essential tips to keep in mind:

Maintain alignment: Pay close attention to your body's alignment during each exercise. Keep your spine neutral, your shoulders relaxed, and your core muscles engaged to support your movements.

Mindful breathing: Remember to breathe steadily and rhythmically throughout each exercise. Your breath not only fuels your movements but also helps maintain focus and prevent unnecessary tension.

Start slowly and gradually: If you're new to Wall Pilates, begin with the basic exercises and progress at your own pace. Avoid rushing through movements; instead, focus on controlled and precise execution.

Use proper footwear: Wear comfortable, supportive footwear that provides stability and traction, especially if you're doing weight-bearing exercises. This will help prevent slips or falls.

Listen to your body: Pay attention to any discomfort or pain. If you experience sharp or persistent pain during an exercise, stop and reassess your form. Consult a healthcare professional if needed.

Utilize props safely: If you're incorporating props like resistance bands or balls, ensure they are secure and used as directed. Improper use can lead to accidents or strain.

Stay hydrated: Maintain proper hydration before, during, and after your Wall Pilates session. Dehydration can affect your performance and increase the risk of muscle cramps.

Seek professional guidance: If you're uncertain about a particular exercise or technique, consider working with a certified Pilates instructor. They can provide personalized guidance and ensure you're performing exercises correctly.

Warm-up and cool-down: Pilates Always begin your session with a gentle warm-up to prepare your body for exercise. Likewise, end with a cool-down to gradually lower your heart rate and stretch out your muscles.

Be consistent: Consistency is key to progress but avoid over-training. Listen to your body's signals and allow for adequate rest and recovery between sessions.

MINDFULNESS AND EMOTIONAL WELL-BEING: MORE THAN MUSCLE

In my early years, I held the belief that the gym was a place solely for sculpting muscles and enhancing physical allure. While that notion holds some truth, as I matured, I came to understand that strength training embodies so much more than the pursuit of bulging biceps.

I vividly recall a pivotal moment from a few years ago when both my career and personal life hit a rough patch. It felt as though the world had lost its coherence, and I found myself grappling with a profound sense of discontent. It was during this challenging juncture that a dear friend of mine extended a simple yet transformative invitation. "You've weathered this storm for quite some time," he remarked, "why not join me at the gym and let off some steam?"

Though skeptical of how lifting weights could alleviate my emotional burdens, I decided to give it a try. That single session marked the inception of a new sanctuary in my life. Now, whenever life serves up its share of stressors, my instinctive refuge is strength training. There, amidst the clinking of weights and the rhythm of my breath, I find solace and renewal.

These years of faithful commitment to strength training have profoundly altered my outlook on life. It's not merely about physicality; it's about fortifying the mind and soul. Today, I stand as a testament to the extraordinary impact that strength training can have on one's mentality and self-assurance. It's a journey that transcends the superficial, a journey that has empowered me in ways I could have never imagined.

Strength training is a testament to your inner fortitude. It requires dedication, consistency, and a willingness to push past perceived limitations. As you witness your physical strength grow, so too does your mental resilience. You learn that challenges are not insurmountable obstacles but rather opportunities for growth and transformation.

Each repetition, each set, is a testament to your ability to persevere. It teaches you that you are capable of far more than you initially believed. This newfound mental resilience permeates other areas of your life, bolstering your confidence in facing challenges beyond the realm of Wall Pilates.

With each milestone reached in your strength training journey, you'll find a surge in self-confidence. It's not just about physical appearance but rather a deep-seated belief in your own capabilities. You stand taller, not only because of the physical strength you've gained but also because of your inner knowing that you are capable and strong.

This confidence transcends the gym or your Wall Pilates practice. It seeps into your daily life, influencing how you approach tasks, interact with others, and navigate challenges. You carry yourself with a sense of assurance, knowing that you have the inner and outer strength to face whatever comes your way.

Strength training is a powerful union of mind and body. It teaches you that true strength is not just about physical might but also about the resilience and confidence that emanate from within. It's a reminder that you are not defined by external circumstances but rather by the inner fire that propels you forward.

Mindful Muscle Engagement

As earlier mentioned, strength training brings the mind and body to equilibrium and incorporating mindfulness into strength training further deepens this mind-body connection. Here is how you can infuse mindfulness into your strength training sessions:

Set your intention: Before you begin an exercise, take a moment to set a clear intention. Focus on what you aim to achieve, not just physically but also mentally and emotionally. This could be a feeling of strength, resilience, or accomplishment.

Conscious breath: As you approach the exercise, bring your attention to your breath. Take a few slow, deliberate breaths, inhaling deeply through your nose and exhaling slowly through your mouth. Feel the rhythm of your breath grounding you in the present moment.

Engage with awareness: As you perform the exercise, pay close attention to the specific muscle groups involved. Visualize the muscles contracting and releasing with each movement. Tune into the sensations, noticing the warmth, tension, and energy flow.

Maintain presence: Avoid letting your mind wander. If you notice distractions or thoughts arising, gently guide your focus back to the exercise and your breath. This practice of returning to the present moment builds mental resilience.

Reflect on strength: After completing the exercise, take a moment to reflect on the strength you've just demonstrated. Acknowledge the progress, no matter how small. Feel a sense of gratitude for your body's capabilities.

This mindful approach to strength training not only enhances the effectiveness of your exercises but also cultivates a deeper sense of connection with your body.

FROM SKEPTIC TO STRENGTH: BRYAN'S REMARKABLE PILATES JOURNEY

Meet Bryan Wilson, a 64-year-old carpenter and musician whose life has been transformed through Wall Pilates at Moving Spirit Studio. Bryan's initial skepticism about Pilates, stemming from the misconception that it was primarily for appearance rather than tangible benefits, kept him away for over 25 years. However, as the physical demands of his carpentry work began to take a toll on his body, Bryan decided to give Pilates another chance.

Despite trying conventional approaches like weightlifting, videos, and outdoor activities, Bryan's joints continued to ache, and certain movements were off-limits due to fear of injury. Even with his wife being a seasoned Pilates instructor, Bryan's prior negative experience with a mat class left him hesitant.

Upon starting Pilates, Bryan was surprised at how deceptively gentle the exercises seemed. However, he soon noticed positive changes. His body felt looser, and he moved with greater ease.

Over time, Bryan's strength and mobility improved significantly. He found himself more energetic and less uncomfortable in his daily activities.

Pilates offered Bryan a level of specificity and technique that differed from his previous workouts. It focused on working deeper muscles, leading to increased strength and reduced joint pain. Bryan's once bulky muscles became leaner yet significantly stronger. His newfound mobility allowed him to move confidently, without the need for strategizing or bracing to prevent injury.

Through Pilates, Bryan not only regained physical vitality but also experienced a profound shift in how he perceived and moved through the world. It wasn't just an exercise; it was a transformative journey toward a more vibrant, energetic, and confident version of himself (Steers, 2020).

This story emphasizes how Pilates, specifically Wall Pilates, can provide tangible, life-changing benefits, especially for individuals with physically demanding occupations like carpentry. It underscores that Pilates is not just about aesthetics but about functional strength and well-being.

NUTRITION TIPS FOR STRENGTH TRAINING

Nutrition plays a vital role in supporting your muscle-building journey. Here are some foods and drinks that are particularly beneficial for building muscle and aiding in recovery:

Lean proteins: Incorporate lean sources of protein like chicken, turkey, fish, lean beef, and tofu. These provide the essential building blocks for muscle repair and growth.

Complex carbohydrates: Choose complex carbohydrates such as whole grains (brown rice, quinoa), and sweet potatoes. These are crucial for replenishing glycogen stores and providing energy during workouts.

Healthy fats: Include sources like avocados, nuts, and seeds. They provide sustained energy and support overall health.

Leafy greens and vegetables: Load up on a variety of colorful vegetables and leafy greens. They are rich in essential vitamins, minerals, and antioxidants that aid in recovery and overall well-being.

Dairy or plant-based alternatives: Greek yogurt and their plant-based counterparts are excellent sources of protein and calcium, which are essential for muscle health.

Supplements: If needed, consider supplements like protein powders, BCAAs (Branched-Chain Amino Acids), and creatine. Consult a healthcare professional before adding supplements to your diet.

Congratulations on investing in your strength and well-being through proper nutrition! You've taken a significant step toward achieving your fitness goals.

As you've discovered, the right nutrition fuels your body, aiding in muscle growth and recovery. But that's not where our journey ends. In fact, it's just the beginning.

In the next chapter, we'll delve into the intriguing connection between physical and mental strength. You'll explore how a strong body can contribute to a resilient mind, and vice versa. It's an exciting continuation of your path toward holistic well-being.

7

MIND-BODY CONNECTION

H ave you ever experienced a moment where your body moved in perfect harmony with your thoughts? Where every motion feels effortless, and every breath aligns with intention? This is the essence of the mind-body connection.

The mind-body connection is a profound synergy between your mental and physical states. It's the art of being fully present in your movements, of feeling every muscle engagement, and of understanding the subtleties of your body's responses. Imagine a seamless dance between your mind's intentions and your body's execution.

In Wall Pilates, this connection is paramount. It transforms your practice from a series of exercises into a holistic experience. It's more than just physical exertion; it's a mindful journey that engages your entire being.

Why is this connection crucial in Wall Pilates, you ask? It's the secret to unlocking the full potential of your practice. When you cultivate a strong mind-body link, you enhance your ability to lower stress levels, improve focus, and elevate your overall performance. It's the difference between merely going through the motions and experiencing a transformative, whole-body engagement.

As we delve deeper into this chapter, we'll explore techniques and practices to strengthen this invaluable connection. Get ready to embark on a journey that transcends the physical, leading to a more profound and enriching Wall Pilates experience.

PROGRESSIVE EXERCISES: CONNECT YOUR MIND AND MUSCLES

Wall Squat Mindfulness

- Stand against the wall with your feet hip-width apart.
- With your back against the wall and feet planted firmly, start to lower your body into a squat position. As you descend, pay close attention to the sensations in your body. Feel the engagement in your leg muscles and the gradual bending of your knees.
- Hold for five breaths. As you maintain your posture, continue to concentrate on your breath. Each inhale and exhale serves to anchor you in the present moment, fostering a sense of mindfulness.

- Return to standing. As you ascend, feel the muscles in your legs working in unison to straighten your body.

This exercise invites you to truly inhabit each moment of the movement. Feel the steady support of the wall against your back, and let your breath guide you through the squat. Notice the subtle shifts in your body as you hold the position. This exercise lays a strong foundation for the mind-body connection in your Wall Pilates practice.

One-Leg Balance with Deep Breathing

This particular movement is not only about physical stability but also about cultivating a deep sense of inner calm and focus.

- Begin by standing tall with your feet hip-width apart. Take a moment to ground yourself, feeling the weight evenly distributed between both feet.
- Slowly shift your weight onto your right leg, gently lifting your left foot off the ground. Bring your hands to your hips for added support.
- Fix your gaze on a steady point in front of you. This will help you maintain balance and concentration throughout the exercise.
- As you find your balance, take a slow and deep inhalation through your nose. Feel your chest and abdomen expand with the breath.
- Gradually exhale through your mouth, allowing any tension to release. Feel a sense of grounding and stability in your standing leg.

- Maintain this posture for about 5-7 breaths, continuing to breathe deeply and steadily.
- Gently lower your lifted leg and shift your weight onto it while raising the opposite foot. Repeat the process on the other side.

This exercise not only strengthens your physical balance but also nurtures your mental focus and breath awareness. It's a beautiful fusion of stability and mindfulness.

Wall Push-Up with Breath Counting

- Stand facing the wall with your arms extended and your palms flat against the wall at shoulder height. Your feet should be about hip-width apart, and your body should form a straight line from head to heels.
- Ensure your body forms a straight line from head to heels. Engage your core muscles for stability.
- Take a slow, deep breath in through your nose as you begin to bend your elbows, lowering your chest toward the wall.
- Exhale slowly through your mouth as you push away from the wall, straightening your arms. Imagine pushing the wall away from you.
- After each push, take a moment to count your breaths. Inhale and exhale for a count of four or choose a breath count that feels comfortable for you.
- Continue the push-up motion, synchronized with your breath count. Focus on smooth, controlled movements.

- Aim for 8–10 repetitions or adjust based on your
  current level of strength and comfort.

This exercise not only targets your upper-body strength but
also encourages mindful breathing. The breath counting adds a
rhythmic element, helping to sync your breath with your
movements.

Wall Plank to Engage Core and Mind

This dynamic movement not only strengthens your core but
also fosters a deep connection between your mind and body.

- Stand facing the wall, about an arm's length away. Place
  your hands on the wall at shoulder height, shoulder-
  width apart. Step your feet back, creating a straight line
  from head to heels.
- Imagine drawing your belly button toward your spine.
  This action engages your core muscles, providing
  stability and support.
- Focus on keeping your body in a straight line, like a
  plank. Avoid letting your hips sag or raising them too
  high.
- Take slow, deep breaths as you hold the plank position.
  Inhale through your nose, and exhale through your
  mouth.
- Aim to hold the wall plank for 20–30 seconds initially.
  As you progress, you can increase the duration.

- While holding the plank, concentrate on the sensations in your body. Feel the engagement of your core, the strength in your arms, and the stability in your legs.
- Imagine yourself becoming stronger with each breath. Picture the energy flowing through your body, reinforcing your core.
- When you're ready to finish, gently step your feet back toward the wall and stand upright.

Remember, quality is more important than quantity. Focus on maintaining proper form and alignment throughout the exercise.

By combining core engagement with mindful breathing, you're nurturing the essential connection between your mind and body. This practice is at the heart of Wall Pilates, promoting both physical strength and mental clarity.

Standing Leg Lifts for Focus and Control

- Begin by standing tall with your feet hip-width apart. Find a point in front of you to focus on, aiding in balance and concentration.
- Gently draw your belly button toward your spine to activate your core muscles. This stabilizes your body and prepares you for the movement.
- Slowly raise one leg straight in front of you. Keep it extended and parallel to the ground. Hold this position for a moment.

- Focus on keeping your lifted leg steady and controlled. Avoid any sudden, jerky movements.
- As you hold the leg lift, take steady breaths in and out. This conscious breathing enhances your focus and maintains a calm state of mind.
- Imagine a line of energy running from the crown of your head down through your standing leg and out through your lifted foot. This mental image helps with balance.
- Lower your lifted leg back to the ground with control, and then repeat the movement with the opposite leg.
- Ensure you give both legs equal attention to maintain balance and symmetry.
- As you become more comfortable with this exercise, you can extend the duration of the leg lift or add ankle weights for added resistance.

MINDFULNESS AND EMOTIONAL WELL-BEING: MORE THAN JUST EXERCISE

When you do Wall Pilates with a focused mind, it's like taking a special journey inside yourself. You pay close attention to how your body moves and reacts. It's a bit like exploring the details of a delicate dance.

This deep awareness lets you spot areas of tension, both in your body and in your thoughts. These are like little knots of stress that have built up over time, making your muscles tight or your mind race. By breathing slowly and moving with control, you gently start to untangle these knots. It's like easing out knots in a shoelace, letting the built-up pressure go.

As this happens, something amazing occurs. The stress knots start to relax, and you're left with a wonderful feeling of calm. It's like a gentle wave washing over you, carrying away any left-over tension. This calm feeling isn't just for a moment; it stays with you long after you're done.

And here's something else. Paying such close attention to your body's movements naturally helps you ignore outside distractions. The noise and busyness of the world fade away. Your mind, now tuned into your breathing and movements, creates a quiet and peaceful place. Within this peaceful place, the chaos of the outside world can't bother you.

In this calm space, stress has a hard time bothering you. It's a place where worries disappear, replaced by a calm feeling of being right here, right now. It's like a safe space you carry with you—a haven from the everyday rush. Through Wall Pilates and this mindful connection, you've found a way to have lasting calm and a shield against the stresses of the outside world.

Additional Mindfulness Tips

Intentional presence: Imagine your Wall Pilates practice as a sacred moment of connection between your mind and body. Intentional presence is about wholeheartedly immersing yourself in this experience. It's a conscious choice to be fully present, both mentally and physically, in every single movement.

As you engage in each exercise, bring your focus to the minutiae of the process. Feel the subtleties of muscle engagement; notice how each fiber awakens and contributes to the motion. It's akin to a symphony where each instrument plays a unique role, creating a harmonious composition. Similarly, every muscle in your body plays a crucial part in the graceful flow of movement.

Sensory awareness: Sensory awareness means paying close attention to how your body feels during your exercises. It's like having a conversation with your body. You're listening to the gentle stretches, the firm muscles, and the rhythm of your breath. This helps you understand and appreciate how amazing your body is at sensing and adapting to movement.

When you practice sensory awareness, you're choosing to be fully present in the moment. It's like appreciating a beautiful painting, but instead, you're appreciating the feelings inside your body. This practice helps you become more connected with your body. It's like becoming good friends with yourself. This connection doesn't stop after your exercise; it carries over into your everyday life. You'll find yourself more aware of your body and how it feels, even outside of your exercise routine.

Embrace imperfection: Embracing imperfection in Wall Pilates means understanding that progress takes time and practice. It's like learning a new move; you might not get it right on the first try. Give yourself the space to learn and grow without being too hard on yourself. Don't judge your early attempts too harshly. Remember, it's all part of the journey toward mastering the exercises.

For instance, when you first attempt a challenging Wall Pilates posture, it's normal to feel a bit unsteady or struggle to maintain proper form. Instead of getting discouraged, remind yourself that it's part of the learning process. With consistent practice and patience, you'll gradually improve and perform the move with confidence and precision.

Gratitude practice: Practicing gratitude in Wall Pilates involves taking a moment, either before or after your session, to appreciate what your body can do. This simple act of acknowledging your body's capabilities can have a powerful impact on your mindset. It cultivates a positive outlook, helping you approach your practice with a sense of appreciation and encouragement.

Visualize your goals: When engaging in certain exercises, take a moment to visualize the strength and balance you aspire to attain. Picture yourself achieving these goals in your mind. This mental imagery can have a powerful effect, enhancing your physical performance and helping you move closer to realizing your objectives.

Release tension with breath: If you feel any tension building up, take a deliberate exhale and visualize it leaving your body with your breath. This simple practice can help you let go of any unwanted tension and promote a sense of relaxation.

Transition mindfully: Transitioning mindfully means taking the sense of awareness and presence you cultivate during your Wall Pilates practice and carrying it with you into your everyday life. As you move through your day, pay attention to how this mindfulness enhances your interactions and experiences. You might find that you're more focused, present, and engaged in each moment. This can lead to deeper connections with others, a greater appreciation for the little things, and an overall sense of fulfillment in your daily activities. It's a way to infuse mindfulness into every aspect of your life, creating a more meaningful and enriching experience.

BENEFITS OF A STRONG MIND-BODY CONNECTION

Building a strong mind-body connection through Wall Pilates offers a range of powerful benefits. Let's delve into how this connection can positively impact your overall well-being.

Enhanced physical performance: When your mind and body work together seamlessly, you unlock a new level of physical potential. Movements become more fluid, controlled, and efficient. You'll notice improved posture, balance, and coordination.

Reduced stress and anxiety: A strong mind-body connection allows you to be present in the moment. This mindfulness practice helps calm the whirlwind of thoughts, reducing stress and anxiety. It's like a sanctuary of peace in the midst of life's demands.

Improved focus and concentration: As you train your mind to be present in every movement, you're also training it to focus. This newfound mental discipline extends beyond your practice and into your daily life, enhancing your ability to concentrate on tasks.

Greater emotional resilience: The mind-body connection nurtures emotional well-being. It provides a toolset to navigate through challenges with grace and stability. You'll find that you're better equipped to handle stressful situations and maintain a positive outlook.

Heightened body awareness: Through Wall Pilates, you'll develop an acute awareness of your body's signals. You'll recognize areas of tension, discomfort, or imbalance, allowing for targeted self-care and prevention of potential issues (Ward, 2023).

Long-lasting calmness: The calmness cultivated through this practice doesn't fade quickly. It's a lasting state of inner peace that accompanies you long after your session ends. This tranquility acts as a shield against the chaos of the outside world.

Improved mindfulness in daily life: The skills you acquire in Wall Pilates spill over into your everyday activities. You'll find yourself more mindful, present, and engaged in your day-to-day experiences, leading to a richer, more fulfilling life.

NUTRITION TIPS: EAT FOR YOUR BRAIN

Nourishing your brain is just as important as strengthening your body. Incorporating certain foods into your diet can have a profound impact on your cognitive function and overall well-being. Here are some brain-boosting foods you might want to consider:

Fatty fish: Fish like salmon, trout, and sardines are rich in omega-3 fatty acids. These healthy fats are essential for brain health and can enhance cognitive function.

Leafy greens: Vegetables like spinach, kale, and Swiss chard are packed with nutrients like folate, vitamin K, and antioxidants. These elements support brain health and help protect against cognitive decline.

Berries: Blueberries, strawberries, and other berries are high in antioxidants, which may delay brain aging and improve memory.

Nuts and seeds: Almonds, walnuts, flaxseeds, and chia seeds are excellent sources of nutrients that benefit brain health. They contain omega-3 fatty acids, antioxidants, and vitamin E.

Avocados: This fruit is a great source of healthy fats, vitamin K, and folate, which are all beneficial for brain health.

Turmeric: The active ingredient in turmeric, called curcumin, has been shown to cross the blood-brain barrier and has anti-inflammatory and antioxidant benefits. It may also boost brain levels of brain-derived neurotrophic factor (BDNF), a growth hormone that functions in the brain.

Now, how do these foods tie into Wall Pilates? Well, a nourished brain complements a focused and mindful practice. When your brain is well fed, you're likely to experience increased concentration, improved memory, and enhanced mental clarity during your Pilates sessions. This means you can fully engage with each movement, getting the most out of your practice.

Now that we've delved into the profound connection between your mind and body, it's time to shift our focus to the mental aspect of Wall Pilates. In the next chapter, we'll guide you on customizing your workout to maximize its benefits and amplify your enjoyment of this transformative practice. Get ready to unlock the full potential of your Wall Pilates journey!

8

CUSTOMIZATION

L et's start with a fundamental truth: When it comes to Wall Pilates, there's no one-size-fits-all approach. You might have come across advice insisting, "This is the routine to follow," leaving you questioning if you've been on the wrong path. Allow me to ease your mind: The most effective Wall Pilates routine is the one that resonates with you.

Reflecting on my own journey into wall Pilates a few years ago, I vividly recall immersing myself in countless YouTube videos, diligently following the routines laid out by various instructors. While these videos did help in perfecting the steps, I soon realized that my mind and body were yearning for something different. That's when I decided to forge my own path, crafting a routine that aligned with how I wanted my mind and body to feel.

In the initial days, it was a challenge, no doubt. Yet, with each passing day, I settled into it, fine-tuning my routine as my practice advanced. The beauty of this journey was the space it offered for growth and experimentation. I tailored my workouts to suit my preferences and cater to my unique needs.

This is the essence of Wall Pilates—a canvas where you paint your own masterpiece. It's about moving your body in ways that feel right to you, ways that elevate your emotional well-being. In this chapter, our aim is to provide you with the guidance to customize your Wall Pilates practice.

PROGRESSIVE EXERCISES

In this transformative section, we'll embark on a journey from fundamental to intermediate and, finally, to the pinnacle of advanced exercises. These carefully curated movements are designed not only to fortify your physical prowess but also to cultivate unwavering determination and unyielding resilience.

Wall Push-Up

Basic Wall Push-Up

- Stand an arm's length away from the wall, feet shoulder-width apart.
- Place your hands flat on the wall, slightly wider than shoulder-width, at chest level.
- Engage your core and maintain a straight line from head to heels.
- Slowly bend your elbows, lowering your body towards the wall.

- Push back to the starting position, fully extending your arms.

Intermediate Wall Push-Up

- Take a step back from the wall, creating a slight angle.
- Follow the same steps as the basic push-up, ensuring your body remains aligned.
- Feel the increased challenge in your arms and chest.

Advanced Wall Push-Up (with Leg Lift)

- Step further back from the wall to intensify the exercise.
- Lift one leg off the ground, keeping it straight and in line with your body.
- Perform the push-up as before, maintaining balance with one leg raised.
- Alternate legs for each repetition.

Wall Squat

Basic Wall Squat

- Stand tall with your back against the wall, feet shoulder-width apart.
- Slowly slide down the wall, bending your knees until they form a 90-degree angle.
- Push through your heels, rising back up to the starting position.

Intermediate Wall Squat

- Follow the steps for the basic squat.
- Once at the 90-degree position, hold the squat for a few invigorating seconds.
- Feel the burn and the strengthening power surge through your legs.

Advanced Wall Squat (with Leg Lift)

- Embrace the challenge by holding the squat position.
- Elevate your practice by adding a leg lift while in the squat.
- Feel the graceful balance and strength that courses through you.

Wall Tap

Basic Wall Tap

- Stand a few inches from the wall, feet hip-width apart.
- Extend your arms and gently tap the wall with your fingertips.
- Feel the connection, the energy flowing through you.

Intermediate Wall Tap

- Step a bit further back from the wall.
- With determination in your step, extend your arms and tap the wall.

- Experience the subtle shift and the growing confidence in your movements.

Advanced Wall Tap (on One Leg)

- Elevate your practice by balancing on one leg.
- With unwavering focus, extend your arms and tap the wall.
- Sense the power, the harmony between body and mind.

Wall Plank

Basic Wall Plank

- Gently lean into the wall, supporting yourself with your forearms.
- Feel the stability and foundation beneath you.

Intermediate Wall Plank

- Take a confident step back to increase the incline.
- Embrace the challenge and the surge of determination.

Advanced Wall Plank (with Alternating Knee Taps)

- Elevate your practice by adding alternating knee taps.
- Experience the flow, the synchronization of movement.

Wall Side Leg Lifts

Basic Wall Side Leg Lifts

- Stand close to the wall, feeling its supportive presence.
- Lift one leg gently to the side, embracing the freedom of movement.

Intermediate Wall Side Leg Lifts

- Hold the lifted leg up for a couple of precious seconds.
- Feel the power and grace radiate through you.

Advanced Wall Side Leg Lifts (with Ankle Weight)

- Elevate your practice by adding an ankle weight.
- Embrace the challenge, the exhilaration of progress.

It's not about achieving perfection in every movement. It's about embracing the challenge and celebrating your progress, no matter the level. As you embark on these exercises, listen to your body. Feel the strength coursing through you and know that every effort counts.

CUSTOMIZATION TIPS

Embracing the power of customization in your Wall Pilates journey is a profound act of self-care and self-discovery. It's a declaration that your practice is uniquely yours, tailored to meet you exactly where you are, physically and emotionally.

When you customize your routine, you grant yourself the gift of adaptability. You have the freedom to choose exercises that resonate with you, that speak to your body's needs and desires. This personal touch transforms your practice into a sanctuary, a sacred space where you can explore, grow, and heal.

Moreover, customization empowers you to set and achieve meaningful goals. It allows you to progress at your own pace, celebrating each milestone along the way. This sense of accomplishment becomes a wellspring of confidence, not just in your practice, but in every aspect of your life.

Through customization, you unlock the true potential of Wall Pilates. It becomes more than a physical exercise; it becomes a holistic practice that nurtures your mind, body, and spirit. It's an intimate dialogue between you and the wall, a dance of strength, grace, and resilience.

Customizing your Wall Pilates routine is like tailoring a suit; it ensures a perfect fit for your unique needs and aspirations. Here are some heartfelt tips to help you sculpt a practice that feels just right for you:

Adjust Your Distance from the Wall

Throughout this practice, the wall is your steadfast ally toward self-discovery through Wall Pilates. The distance you choose from it holds the key to a tailored experience just for you.

When you stand closer, it's like a reassuring hand on your back, offering a comforting embrace. This proximity provides a stable foundation, allowing you to explore each movement with confidence. It's akin to having a trusted friend by your side, ensuring you feel supported and secure.

Now, should you choose to step back, it's as if you're venturing into the open sea, ready to embrace the challenge. This subtle shift transforms the exercise into a dynamic dance, demanding more from your muscles. It's an invitation to tap into reservoirs of strength you might not have known existed. With each controlled movement, you forge a deeper connection with the reservoirs of power within you.

Mindful Breathwork

As you stand before the wall, consider your breath as your guide. Inhale deeply, drawing in strength and intention, envisioning the adjustments you'll make to suit your needs. Feel the possibilities fill you, just like the canvas waiting for the artist's touch.

With each exhale, let go of any doubts, or hesitations. Picture them dissolving, replaced by a newfound confidence. This is your moment of creation, your customization. As the breath flows, so do the tailored choices, shaping your practice into a masterpiece that resonates with you.

Add or Remove Props

Consider the props as your companions on this artistic journey. When you invite resistance bands or ankle weights, you're infusing the spirit of challenge and vigor into your practice.

Feel the power surge through you, like an artist wielding bold strokes.

Conversely, when you choose to remove these props, it's akin to stepping into a serene, tranquil landscape. Your practice becomes a dance, fluid and gentle, allowing for a deeper connection with your body. It's like an artist using delicate brushwork to bring forth grace and ease.

Modify Your Duration

Imagine our Wall Pilates practice as a beautifully composed melody, with time as our wise conductor, guiding our every move. In this symphony, you are the maestro, holding the baton of control, attuned to the tempo that resonates with your heart's desires.

When you yearn for a gentle embrace, a shorter duration wraps around you like a soft lullaby, cradling your muscles in serene repose. It's a tender moment of respite, allowing your body to find solace in stillness.

Yet, when the call for strength and endurance arises, a longer hold becomes your anthem. With each passing beat, you'll sense your power growing, your spirit ascending to new heights.

Embrace Your Body's Wisdom

Tune in to what your body is telling you. If a certain adjustment feels right, trust that instinct.

Conversely, if something doesn't feel comfortable, don't hesitate to modify it. Your intuition is your wisest guide.

NUTRITION TIPS

Embracing customization in your nutrition plan empowers you to craft a diet that aligns perfectly with your unique preferences and dietary needs. This approach allows you the freedom to select from various food groups, ensuring they adhere to the recommended guidelines for a balanced and nourishing diet.

Imagine curating meals that not only cater to your taste buds but also fuel your body in a way that resonates with your individual goals and aspirations. This level of personalization grants you the opportunity to explore a wide array of options, from lean proteins like poultry and tofu to complex carbohydrates such as quinoa and whole grains.

By incorporating an assortment of colorful fruits and vegetables, you infuse your diet with a diverse range of essential vitamins, minerals, and antioxidants. This vibrant palette not only tantalizes your senses but also provides a robust foundation for overall well-being.

The power of customization lies in your hands. You have the ability to choose combinations that resonate with you, ensuring your dietary journey is not only effective but also enjoyable. So, whether you lean towards plant-based options or embrace a balance of various food groups, the key lies in crafting a plan that speaks to your unique needs.

It's essential to maintain awareness of portion sizes and balance. This ensures you're getting the right mix of nutrients while avoiding overindulgence. Consulting with a healthcare professional or nutritionist can be immensely beneficial in tailoring a plan that harmonizes with your specific requirements.

Ultimately, the beauty of customization in nutrition lies in its adaptability. As you progress on your journey towards a healthier, stronger you, don't hesitate to tweak and refine your approach. After all, it's about finding what works best for you, guiding you towards a path of sustained well-being and vitality.

You're on the brink of something truly transformative. The next chapter is poised to unveil how the magic of Wall Pilates extends far beyond the practice itself, seeping into the tapestry of your daily life.

Get ready to witness how the strength you're nurturing within these sessions will soon become an unshakable foundation, supporting you through every twist and turn. Your journey is about to take an even more extraordinary turn.

9

FUNCTIONAL FITNESS

Functional fitness is more than just a term; it's a key that unlocks the door to a life of ease and vitality. It's about preparing your body to handle daily tasks with grace and vigor. And for those of us who have walked more miles, seen more sunrises, and gathered more wisdom, it becomes nothing short of vital.

You see, functional fitness is the key that unlocks the door to a life of independence, freedom, and joy. It allows you to relish in the simple pleasures, like effortlessly bending to tie your shoes, playing with your grandchildren, or carrying your groceries with confidence.

As we embrace the passage of time, it's not about merely existing; it's about thriving. It's about savoring each moment and knowing that your body is your ally, ready to support you in every endeavor.

This is the magic of functional fitness—it's the bridge between your Wall Pilates practice and the radiant, fulfilling life you deserve. It's about being present in every moment and cherishing the little victories that come from a body and mind in perfect sync.

As we step into Chapter 9, we're venturing into a realm where Wall Pilates transcends the mat and touches every facet of your life. It's about empowering you to glide through your day with grace, especially for those golden souls who've graced us with their wisdom.

PROGRESSIVE EXERCISES

Progression is the heartbeat of functional fitness. It's the dynamic force that propels us forward, unlocking new levels of strength, balance, and agility. Just as the seasons change and life evolves, so too should our approach to exercise.

Think of it as a journey. You start at one point, but you don't remain there forever. You push boundaries, you challenge yourself, and you grow. Each step you take, whether it's mastering a Wall Push-Up or conquering a Wall Plank with Leg Lifts, is a testament to your dedication to progress.

Embrace this journey, for it's not about perfection, but about growth. As you advance through these exercises, you'll discover newfound capabilities within yourself. What may seem daunting today will become a triumph tomorrow.

Single-Leg Wall Squat

- Stand tall with your back against the wall, feet planted firmly on the ground.
- Lift one leg gently in front of you, finding your balance and holding it there.
- Slowly start sliding down into a squat on the other leg, making sure your knee aligns with your ankle.
- As you lower down, feel the strength in your leg supporting you.
- Hold this position for a moment, breathing steadily and feeling the stability in your body.
- Push through your heel to return to the standing position.
- Switch legs and repeat the motion.

Wall Mountain Climbers

- Position yourself facing the wall, hands firmly planted on it.
- Step back with your feet until you're in a plank position, with your body in a straight line.
- Now, imagine you're scaling a mountain. Bring one knee toward your chest, using your core muscles to draw it in.
- As you return that foot back, bring the other knee up toward your chest.
- Alternate between legs, moving in a controlled and deliberate manner.

- Keep the rhythm steady, feeling the burn in your core and the energy flowing through you.

Wall Plank with Leg Lift

- Position yourself in a strong wall plank, hands firmly on the ground and body forming a straight line.
- Now, lift one leg up gently, feeling the engagement in your core and the strength in your arms.
- Slowly lower the leg back down, maintaining control and stability.
- Switch to the other leg and repeat this uplifting motion.
- Feel the connection between your mind, body, and the support of the wall.

Wall Angels

- Stand tall with your back against the wall, arms extended at shoulder height.
- Begin to slide your arms upwards along the wall, as if you're painting a majestic snow angel in the air.
- Feel the gentle resistance and the graceful extension of your arms.
- Then, slowly bring your arms back down, savoring the controlled descent.
- Repeat this fluid motion, letting it become a dance with the wall.

Side Wall Plank Rotation

- Begin in a side plank, one hand firmly planted against the supporting wall.
- Feel the stability of the wall against your hand, grounding you.
- Gently start to rotate your torso toward the wall, like a graceful turn in a dance.
- Then, with intention, rotate away, letting your body follow the rhythm of your breath.
- Sense the connection between your muscles and the steadfast support of the wall.

Isometric Wall Push

- Gently position your hands on the wall, arms outstretched, ready to embrace the challenge.
- Feel the connection between your palms and the wall— a promise of support.
- Now, with unwavering determination, push against the wall, tapping into the reservoir of strength within.
- Wall Sit with Calf Raise
- Feel the energy surge through your arms—a steady, unwavering force.

Wall Plank Knee Tucks

- Begin in the wall plank position, with your arms solidly supporting your frame. Feel the connection between your palms and the wall, a conduit of strength.

- Let the power of your core surge forth like a beacon of vitality. This is your source of stability, the anchor that holds you steady.
- Inhale deeply, drawing in the essence of fortitude. Feel your chest rise with purpose.
- With intent, bring one knee toward your chest. Imagine it as a salute to your own resilience.
- Pause for a heartbeat. Let the proximity of knee to chest be a testament to your inner might.
- Extend your leg back, restoring the equilibrium of the plank. Each movement is a symphony, a testament to your grace.
- Repeat the process with the other knee, a rhythmic exchange of power and poise.

Wall Supported Single-Leg Deadlift

- Begin by holding onto the wall, a steadfast companion on your journey. Feel its support, a testament to your unyielding determination.
- Raise the opposite leg, like unfurling a banner of strength. It hovers, a symbol of your potential.
- Gently tip your torso forward, a nod to the earth's embrace. Let gravity be your ally, guiding you toward growth.
- As you lean, sense the ground beneath. It cradles you, offering stability and grounding.
- In this poised moment, you are a portrait of balance. Your lifted leg and extended torso form a tableau of tenacity.

- With intention, return to your starting position, a testament to your adaptability. Each movement is a brushstroke, crafting a masterpiece of strength.
- Repeat this dance with the other leg, a duet of determination and grace.

Wall Sit with Arm Circles

- Nestle into the wall sit position, a sanctuary of stability. Feel the support enveloping you—a reassuring embrace.
- Extend your arms like wings ready to take flight. They are the conduits of your power, poised for movement.
- Begin your small, deliberate circles, each rotation a brushstroke of resilience. Forward and onward, you sculpt the air.
- As your arms glide, sense the momentum building. It's the symphony of your strength, a crescendo of determination.
- Shift the circles in reverse, an ode to adaptability. You are the conductor of this movement, guiding it with purpose.
- Even in the wall sit, know that you are in motion. Every second is a testament to your unwavering resolve.
- Merge the stillness and the movement, a duet of poise and power. You are the embodiment of harmony.

EVERYDAY ACTIVITIES MADE EASIER

Imagine a life where every movement flows with grace, where daily tasks become effortless strokes of mastery. This is the promise that Wall Pilates holds for you.

Rising with Grace

Awakening to a new day, imagine Wall Squats as your gentle embrace. They cradle you, coaxing your body to rise with grace. The once arduous task of standing transforms into a fluid motion, a dance with dawn. It's as if your body remembers the rhythm, seamlessly transitioning from slumber's embrace to the confident stride of a new beginning.

Embracing the Heights

It's more than an exercise; it's a key to a new realm of strength. As your arms gain power, so does your ability to conquer heights. Reaching for the highest shelf is no longer a stretch of strain; it's a dance of ease. Your arms, now fortified, elevate you, allowing you to embrace what once felt out of reach. It's a symphony of empowerment, each push-up a note in the melody of newfound capability.

Retrieving Radiance

Envision this scene: You come across a fallen pen, a small task in the grand scheme of things. Yet, with the grace bestowed by Single-Leg Wall Squats, it transforms into a moment of radiance. There's a newfound ease, a dance of balance and strength as you effortlessly retrieve what was once out of reach. It's a testament to the power of tailored exercises, turning ordinary moments into a celebration of capability.

Carrying Life's Burdens

Life presents its burdens, both literal and metaphorical. Yet, armed with the strength cultivated through Wall Planks, you approach them with a newfound grace. Lifting transforms from a daunting task to a harmonious partnership between you and the weight. Your body rises to the occasion, proving itself capable of shouldering life's challenges with poise and resilience.

Nimbly Navigating

Imagine this: With the agility honed through Wall Mountain Climbers, ascending stairs evolves from a mere task into a personal triumph. Each step you take is marked by a newfound confidence and poise, turning what was once ordinary into a testament of your inner strength. It's as if you're dancing up those steps, leaving no doubt that you've unlocked a new level of nimbleness and grace.

Graceful Grabs

With Wall Plank and Leg Lifts, you possess a secret weapon. It transforms seizing an opportunity into an art, executed with finesse and flair. Imagine reaching out, not just with strength, but with a graceful assurance that leaves an indelible mark. This exercise empowers you to grasp life's moments with a touch of elegance, turning each opportunity into a masterpiece of your own creation.

Elegant Extensions

Imagine that you are reaching for that cherished book on the top shelf or effortlessly extending to grab your favorite mug from the cupboard. With the gracefulness nurtured by Wall Angels, these acts become moments of pure artistry.

I remember a time when a senior friend of mine struggled to reach high places, feeling a tug of strain. But now, thanks to Wall Angels, it's a different story. Every reach is a testament to the strength and beauty within. It's not just a physical movement; it's a dance of elegance and strength, and it's yours to embrace.

The Rise of Resilience

Picture this: You, standing tall on one leg, reaching for the sky. It's more than a mere physical act; it's a powerful testament to your unbreakable spirit, a gift from Wall Taps.

I remember when I first attempted this, wobbling and uncertain. But with each tap, I felt my strength grow. Now, it's not just an exercise; it's a statement of my resilience. And it can be yours too. Every tap is a step toward unwavering strength, a reminder that you're capable of more than you know.

NUTRITION TIPS

Muscle Strength

Lean meats: Imagine a succulent piece of grilled chicken or a tender cut of lean beef. These meats are more than just delicious; they're a treasure trove of protein, the fundamental nutrient your muscles thrive on. This high-quality protein provides your body with the essential amino acids it needs to repair and build muscle tissue. It's like giving your muscles the best possible tools to grow stronger and more resilient.

Tofu: You ought to consider tofu, a versatile plant-based marvel. It's not only a rich source of protein but also a complete one, providing your body with all the essential amino acids it requires. This makes tofu an excellent choice for supporting muscle growth and repair. Whether grilled, stir-fried, or blended into smoothies, tofu stands as a reliable plant-powered protein option to fuel your body's strength and vitality.

Beans and legumes: Beans and legumes like black beans, chickpeas, and lentils are exceptional choices. They not only deliver a hearty dose of protein but also come packed with fiber and essential nutrients. This powerful combination is a dynamic force for promoting muscle growth and overall vitality. Whether incorporated into salads, stews, or blended into dips, these humble legumes stand as potent allies in your journey toward a stronger, more vibrant you.

Greek yogurt: Greek yogurt is a creamy delight that's abundant in protein. This makes it an excellent choice for supporting muscle recovery and growth. Enjoy it as a snack or incorporate it into your meals to harness its nourishing benefits.

Balance

Leafy greens: Leafy greens like spinach, kale, and Swiss chard are fantastic additions to your meals. They boast a wealth of vitamins, minerals, and antioxidants, offering a strong foundation for balance. By incorporating these vibrant greens into your diet, you're not only nurturing your body with essential nutrients but also fortifying it for a well-rounded and balanced approach to health.

Colorful fruits: Indulge in a rainbow of fruits, from vibrant berries to juicy oranges and crisp apples. These colorful delights are brimming with essential nutrients that play a crucial role in supporting joint health and overall stability. By relishing in the natural hues of these fruits, you're not only treating your taste buds but also nourishing your body in ways that contribute to a strong and balanced foundation for overall well-being.

Whole Grains: Choose quinoa, brown rice, or whole wheat bread. These choices provide a steady supply of energy, giving you the assurance of staying steadfast on your feet throughout the day. By incorporating these nutritious options into your meals, you're not only savoring their delicious flavors but also fortifying your body with the enduring vitality it craves.

Nuts and seeds: Integrate the natural powerhouses of nutrition into your diet; almonds, chia seeds, or flaxseeds. These little wonders are akin to nature's own energy boosters, providing your body with vital fatty acids that support joint health. By incorporating these wholesome options into your meals, you're not only relishing their rich flavors but also gifting your body the strength and resilience it deserves.

As we conclude this transformative chapter on functional fitness, it's clear that Wall Pilates isn't merely an exercise; it's a gateway to a more vibrant, empowered daily life.

Through these exercises, we've unlocked a world where mundane tasks become graceful movements, and challenges become triumphs. From rising with grace to carrying life's burdens, you've witnessed the magic of functional fitness in action.

Remember that Wall Pilates isn't confined to solitary practice. While you can embark on this journey alone, a community can amplify your progress. It's a haven of shared experiences, mutual support, and boundless motivation.

So, as you step forward into this new realm of functional fitness, know that you're not alone. You're part of a community of fellow seekers, each one on their own path toward strength, balance, and vitality. Together, we'll inspire and lift one another to new heights. Onward we go, hand in hand, toward a life imbued with grace and resilience.

10

COMMUNITY AND SUPPORT

Allow me to introduce you to Harry, a dedicated practitioner of Wall Pilates. He was no stranger to the benefits and challenges that came with this practice. Harry had been navigating his Wall Pilates journey on his own, finding comfort and solace in the rhythm of his practice against the wall.

One day, as the seasons changed and leaves painted the landscape, Harry stumbled upon a vibrant community of fellow Wall Pilates enthusiasts. It was a fortuitous encounter that would profoundly impact his journey.

This newfound community welcomed Harry with open arms. They exchanged stories, techniques, and, most importantly, boundless encouragement. As days turned into weeks, Harry discovered a wellspring of support that propelled him through every practice. The camaraderie fueled his determination, and the shared experiences forged a strong bond.

Together, they celebrated small victories and helped one another overcome challenges. The encouragement extended far beyond physical strength; it was a symphony of emotional fortitude. In moments of doubt, Harry found himself leaning on this newfound family, drawing strength from their collective resolve.

Through this community, Wall Pilates evolved into more than just exercise. It transformed into a shared journey of growth, resilience, and mutual empowerment. The walls that once stood solitary now echoed with laughter, stories, and a symphony of breaths moving in unison.

As you delve into this chapter, remember that you're not alone on this path. The power of community and support is a guiding light that can illuminate even the darkest corners of your journey. Together, we'll explore how being part of a Wall Pilates community can be the root of your success, offering both practical and emotional sustenance. So, let's step forward, hand in hand, into this world of shared strength and unwavering support.

THE POWER OF COMMUNITY

Embarking on a journey, especially one of self-improvement and growth, can sometimes feel like a solitary endeavor. Yet, there's immense power in realizing that you're not alone on this path. That's where community steps in, becoming your steadfast companion, your wellspring of encouragement, and a treasure trove of invaluable tips and wisdom.

In today's interconnected world, communities thrive both in the physical realm and the digital landscape. Let's explore how being part of such a community can elevate your Wall Pilates journey:

SHARED WISDOM AND INSIGHTS

In a community, everyone brings something special to share, like different colors in a woven picture. Each person has their own experiences and clever ideas about Wall Pilates. Some might know little tricks that make exercises work better, while others have calming breathing methods. They're happy to share because they know it can help others.

For example, one person might show a small change in how you stand that makes an exercise much better. Another might teach a breathing trick that makes you more focused and calm. These little bits of wisdom can make your practice go from good to really great.

It's like when friends bring different dishes to a meal. Some might give tips about how to stand or move, while others have ways to make your mind clear and focused. This sharing of ideas makes everyone get better together.

In this group, everyone learns from each other. The shared wisdom is always growing and changing. This keeps the learning going, and everyone gets better because of it. This way of sharing helps everyone in the community grow and get better at Wall Pilates.

UNWAVERING ENCOURAGEMENT

Being part of a community brings a special kind of support. It's like having a team of people who get what you're going through. They celebrate your successes and understand your struggles. This kind of shared encouragement can be a big push forward in your Wall Pilates journey.

Imagine this: You conquer a tough exercise, and your community celebrates with you. Their cheers and applause fill you with a sense of achievement and make you want to do even better. This kind of motivation is like a strong engine that keeps you moving forward in your practice. Knowing that others are there cheering you on can give you that extra boost you need. It's like having your own personal cheering squad!

In this community, everyone understands the challenges and victories because they've been there too. So, when you share your accomplishments, it's met with genuine excitement and support. This kind of encouragement creates a positive atmosphere where everyone feels uplifted and motivated. Together, you become a source of strength for one another, making the journey even more rewarding.

ACCOUNTABILITY AND COMMITMENT

When you're part of a community, it's like having a team that counts on you. You're not just doing it for yourself, but for the whole group. This sense of responsibility can really keep you on track, even when you're not feeling particularly motivated.

Imagine this scenario: It's a day when you're feeling a bit tired or low on energy. Without the support of a community, you might be tempted to skip your Wall Pilates practice. But knowing that others are on this journey with you, counting on you to show up, gives you that extra nudge. It's like having a gentle reminder that every effort you put in matters not just to you, but to the whole community.

This accountability creates a positive cycle. When you commit to a goal alongside others, you're not only answering to yourself, but to the group as a whole. This extra layer of responsibility helps you maintain your dedication, even when the going gets tough. It's like having a friendly push that keeps you moving forward, one step at a time.

ADAPTABILITY AND CUSTOMIZATION

In a community, everyone brings their own unique approach and experiences to the table. It's like a potluck of ideas and insights, each valuable in its own way. This diversity is celebrated and seen as a strength.

For example, let's say there's a particular exercise that some find challenging. Within the community, you might come across different techniques or modifications that individuals have discovered to make it more accessible. This wealth of perspectives opens up a world of possibilities for customizing your practice.

Some might have tips on how to adjust your posture for better alignment, while others might share breathing techniques that enhance focus and relaxation. This diversity of approaches ensures that you have a toolbox of options to tailor your practice to your specific needs.

154 | SEBASTIAN CASTELLANOS

In this way, being part of a community enriches your practice by offering many perspectives and adaptations. It's like having a treasure trove of wisdom at your disposal, allowing you to fine-tune your Wall Pilates journey to align with your individual requirements.

Now, where can you find these communities? They exist in various forms:

Social media: Platforms like Facebook, Reddit, and Instagram have vibrant communities dedicated to fitness, including Wall Pilates. Here, you can connect with enthusiasts, share experiences, and seek advice.

Online forums and groups: Numerous forums and online groups are specifically tailored to Pilates practitioners. These spaces offer a platform for discussions, questions, and the exchange of insights.

Local fitness centers and studios: If you prefer face-to-face interactions, consider joining a local fitness center or Pilates studio. The relationships you build here can be deeply enriching and provide a network of support.

Workshops and classes: Attending workshops or classes in your area is an excellent way to meet fellow practitioners. These events often lead to lasting connections and the opportunity to grow together.

The power of community is a beacon of light, guiding you through every twist and turn. Whether online or in person, these communities offer a sanctuary of support, a treasury of knowledge, and a chorus of encouragement.

STAYING MOTIVATED THROUGH COMMUNITY

When it comes to Wall Pilates, staying motivated is a key to unlocking progress and achieving your goals. And one of the most potent tools at your disposal is the strength of community.

When you're part of a community, setting shared goals or challenges becomes a powerful motivator. Knowing that others are working towards similar milestones can ignite a sense of friendly competition, spurring you to push your boundaries. Celebrating collective triumphs creates a shared sense of achievement, reinforcing your commitment to the practice.

Accountability is a cornerstone of progress. Within a community, this principle takes on a new dimension. When you commit to a goal alongside others, you not only answer to yourself but to the group as a whole. This added layer of accountability can be a powerful force in driving you towards consistency and excellence in your practice.

Picture this: You and your fellow community members embark on a 30-day Wall Pilates challenge. Each day, you share your progress, your triumphs, and even your struggles. The support and encouragement from your peers become a beacon of light, guiding you through every session. On days when motivation wanes, the knowledge that you're not alone in this journey fuels your determination.

In a community, support is woven into every interaction. Whether it's celebrating a new achievement, offering advice on overcoming a hurdle, or simply sharing in the joys and challenges of the practice, the collective energy becomes a source of constant inspiration.

Power of Shared Goals

Firstly, it's important to set goals that are specific, measurable, achievable, relevant, and time-bound. These are often referred to as SMART goals. For instance, instead of a vague goal like "get better at Wall Pilates," aim for something like "improve my balance in Wall Planks by holding the position for an additional 10 seconds by the end of week two."

Next, consider creating goals that align with your personal aspirations. Are you looking to enhance flexibility, build strength, or cultivate mindfulness? Tailor your goals to reflect these intentions. This ensures that your objectives resonate with your individual journey.

Now, let's talk about sharing these goals within your community. This can be done through various channels. If you're part of an online group or forum, consider starting a dedicated thread where members can post their goals and track their progress. In a local studio or fitness center, you might suggest a goal-setting session during community events.

Keep in mind that the key is to create an environment of support and encouragement. When sharing your goals, be open to feedback and suggestions from fellow practitioners. They might offer insights or techniques that you hadn't considered. Likewise, when others share their goals, offer your support and celebrate their achievements, no matter how big or small.

Additionally, consider setting milestones along the way. These are smaller, achievable targets that lead you towards your larger goal. For example, if your main goal is to improve balance on wall planks, a milestone could be adding an extra five seconds to your hold every three days.

Lastly, don't forget to regularly check in with your community about your progress. This can be a weekly update or a monthly reflection. Sharing your successes and any challenges you've faced fosters a sense of accountability and allows your community to provide targeted support and advice.

Here are some techniques and guidelines to help you and your fellow community members set and achieve meaningful goals together:

Open communication: Start by initiating a conversation within the community about setting shared goals. Encourage members to voice their aspirations, challenges, and areas they'd like to focus on in their Wall Pilates practice.

Identify common objectives: Look for common themes or areas of interest that resonate with multiple members. These could range from improving flexibility and balance to mastering specific exercises like wall squats or planks.

Realistic expectations: Set goals that are challenging yet attainable. Consider the collective skill level of the group and avoid setting objectives that might be too advanced for some members.

Time-bound targets: Establish a timeline for achieving the shared goals. This provides a sense of urgency and helps track progress. For instance, aim to achieve a certain milestone within a specified number of weeks.

Break down goals: Divide larger goals into smaller, manageable steps. This makes the process feel less overwhelming and allows for regular check-ins on progress.

Accountability partners: Pair up community members as accountability partners. Encourage them to support and motivate each other in working towards their respective goals.

Regular progress updates: Allocate specific times for members to share their progress. This could be through weekly check-ins or dedicated threads in your community platform.

Celebrate milestones: Acknowledge and celebrate every achievement, no matter how small. This not only boosts morale but also reinforces a culture of support and encouragement.

Adaptability and flexibility: Recognize that individual circumstances may change. Be open to adjusting goals if necessary and provide support for members facing challenges.

Provide constructive feedback: Encourage members to offer constructive feedback to one another. This can include sharing tips, suggesting modifications, or offering words of encouragement.

In this chapter, we've delved into the profound impact of community on your Wall Pilates journey. You've learned how shared goals, accountability, and the tapestry of support can propel you towards greater heights in your practice. Now, it's time to put this knowledge into action.

Introducing the 29-day Wall Pilates Challenge—a journey we're embarking on together. This challenge is not just about physical endurance; it's about cultivating a sense of community and a shared commitment to growth and well-being.

Over the next 29 days, you'll be part of a collective effort, a journey of transformation. We'll celebrate every milestone, overcome every hurdle, and emerge stronger, both individually and as a community.

11

29 DAYS TO A STRONG FOUNDATION

Think of this chapter as your personalized roadmap, guiding you through a metamorphic experience in Wall Pilates. It's more than just a set of exercises; it's a carefully crafted plan that will lead you to a place of profound change and growth.

As you embark on this journey, imagine stepping onto a path that promises not only physical transformation but a deeper connection between your mind and body. This program is designed to be a catalyst for change, setting the stage for a version of yourself that is stronger, more balanced, and in tune with the intricate dance between body and mind.

We're about to embark on a month-long program that will lay the groundwork for a resilient and balanced mind-body connection.

Picture this as the commencement of a 29-day adventure, a dedicated commitment to your own well-being. Each day, you'll be adding a layer of strength, flexibility, and mindfulness to your practice. By the end of this journey, you'll have established a foundation that not only supports your physical endeavors but also nurtures a profound sense of equilibrium between your body and mind.

A strong foundation is the pivot of any successful fitness journey. It provides stability, resilience, and a solid base from which to grow. Over the next 29 days, we'll dive deep into wall Pilates, building strength, enhancing flexibility, and nurturing mental clarity.

Together, we'll progress through carefully designed exercises, each building upon the last, as we work toward a more harmonious and empowered you. By the end of this chapter, you'll not only feel the physical benefits but also carry with you a newfound sense of inner strength.

PHYSICAL HEALTH PROGRESSION: DAY 1 TO DAY 29

Day 1: Foundation Building

Exercise 1: Wall Squats

- Stand against the wall with your feet hip-width apart.
- Lower into a squat while focusing on your breath.
- Hold for five breaths, then return to standing.

Exercise 2: One-Leg Balance with Deep Breathing

- Stand on one leg with a slight bend in the knee.
- Inhale deeply through your nose, allowing your lungs to fill like a gentle breeze.
- Exhale slowly, releasing any tension or resistance.
- Hold for five breaths, then switch legs.

Week 1 Focus (Days 2–7)

Day 2: Wall Push-Ups

- Stand an arm's length away from the wall, with your feet together.
- Place your hands flat against the wall, slightly wider than shoulder-width apart.
- Lower your body toward the wall by bending your elbows.
- Push back to the starting position.
- Tip: Engage your core and maintain a straight line from head to heels throughout the movement.

Day 3: Wall Plank

- Stand facing the wall, arms extended at shoulder height.
- Lean forward, placing your hands on the wall shoulder-width apart.
- Step back with your feet until your body forms a straight line from head to heels.
- Hold this position for 15 seconds.

- Note: Focus on keeping your core engaged and avoid sagging your hips.

Day 4: Wall Taps

- Stand a few inches away from the wall, arms extended at shoulder height.
- Tap the wall with your right hand, then your left hand.
- Continue alternating taps for one minute.
- Reminder: Keep your movements controlled and steady.

Day 5: Wall Mountain Climbers

- Place your hands on the wall, arms extended.
- Step back with your feet into a plank position.
- Bring your right knee toward your chest, then switch to the left, as if climbing a mountain.
- Continue for one minute.
- Important: Maintain a steady pace and engage your core throughout.

Day 6: Wall Plank with Leg Lifts

- Get into a wall plank position.
- Lift your right leg up, then lower it.
- Switch to the left leg.
- Continue alternating for one minute.
- Tip: Focus on stability and controlled leg movements.

Day 7: Wall Supported Single-Leg Deadlift

- Hold onto the wall with your right hand.
- Lift your left leg off the ground while tipping your torso forward.
- Return to the starting position and switch sides.
- Repeat for 10 reps on each leg.

Week 2 Focus (Days 8–14)

Week 2 brings an exciting progression to your Wall Pilates journey. Building on the foundation you've laid, we'll now introduce exercises designed to further enhance your balance, strength, and mindfulness. Add the progressive exercises introduced in Chapter 7.

Day 8: Wall Squat Mindfulness (Progressive Exercise)

- Stand with your back against the wall, feet hip-width apart.
- Slide down into a squat, maintaining the 90-degree angle in your knees.
- Close your eyes and take three slow, deep breaths.
- Focus on the sensations in your body. Notice any areas of tension or ease.
- Tip: Engage your mind in the present moment, appreciating the subtleties of each movement.

Day 9: One-Leg Balance with Deep Breathing (Progressive Exercise)

- Stand with your feet hip-width apart.
- Lift your right foot off the ground, bringing your knee toward your chest.
- Place your hands on your hips and take five deep breaths.
- Repeat on the other leg.
- Reminder: Find a focal point to help with balance and focus on your breath.

Day 10: Wall Push-Up with Breath Counting

- Stand an arm's length away from the wall, hands shoulder-width apart.
- Perform a push-up while inhaling for a count of four.
- Exhale for a count of four as you return to the starting position.
- Note: The breath counting adds a meditative element to this exercise, syncing breath with movement.

Day 11: Wall Plank to Engage Core and Mind

- Get into a wall plank position with your hands on the wall.
- Engage your core and hold for 30 seconds.
- Close your eyes and focus on your breath for another 30 seconds.

- Important: This exercise combines strength and mindfulness, enhancing both physical and mental aspects.

Day 12: Standing Leg Lifts for Focus and Control (Progressive Exercise)

- Stand with your feet together, hands on your hips.
- Lift your right leg in front of you, keeping it straight.
- Hold for 10 seconds, then lower it.
- Repeat with the left leg.
- Tip: This exercise sharpens your focus and strengthens leg muscles.

These exercises, along with the progressive ones introduced in Chapter 7, will be the core of Week 2. Remember to practice daily for 20–25 minutes. Your body and mind will continue to thrive with this balanced routine. Keep up the excellent work!

Week 3 Focus (Days 15–21)

- Continue with the previous exercises and introduce more challenging variations.
- Increase practice time to 30 minutes daily.
- Pay attention to increased ease in performing exercises.

Week 4 Focus (Days 22–29):

- Review and master all exercises from previous weeks.
- Gradually extend practice time to 40 minutes daily.

MEASURING IMPROVEMENT

As you step onto this path of transformative growth, it's essential to have a compass to track your progress. This journey isn't just about going through the motions; it's about observing the evolution, celebrating your victories, and recognizing the subtle shifts that pave the way for lasting change.

When you meticulously note your progress, you're giving yourself the gift of visibility. You'll witness, firsthand, how your body evolves, becoming stronger, more flexible, and more resilient with each passing day. These tangible markers of growth serve as a powerful motivator, reminding you of the incredible strides you're making.

Every individual's journey is unique, and by tracking your progress, you're essentially creating a personalized roadmap. This roadmap is your guide, showing you where you've been and where you're headed. It allows you to identify patterns, areas of strength, and those that may need a bit more attention. This insight is invaluable in tailoring your practice to your specific needs and goals.

Consistency is key in any fitness journey, and measuring improvement reinforces your commitment. It's a visual testament to the effort and dedication you're putting in. On days when motivation might wane, looking back at how far you've come can reignite that spark of determination, propelling you forward.

There's a unique sense of empowerment that comes from tangible evidence of progress. It's a concrete reminder that your efforts are paying off, that the sweat and dedication are yielding real, palpable results. This sense of achievement fuels your confidence, affirming that you're on the right path.

Measuring improvement also sheds light on areas that may require a bit more attention. It's a gentle nudge to explore new techniques, adjust form, or perhaps introduce variations that can further enhance your practice. It's a constructive tool for continuous refinement and growth.

In essence, tracking your progress is like creating a visual diary of your transformation. It's a testament to your commitment, a reflection of your dedication, and a celebration of your growth. So, as you embark on this 29-day journey, remember that each entry in this diary is a testament to your strength, resilience, and unwavering commitment to your own well-being.

Here are some ways to measure your improvement:

Ease of Execution

Proper form: Notice if you're able to maintain the correct posture and alignment more effortlessly. Is your body naturally falling into the prescribed positions? This indicates that your muscles are becoming more accustomed to the movements.

Fluid movements: Observe if the transitions between exercises are smoother. Are you able to flow from one position to the next with greater ease? This suggests improved coordination between your mind and body.

Reduced strain: Pay attention to any signs of strain or tension that you might have initially experienced. Are you feeling less discomfort as you move through the exercises? This is a positive indicator that your muscles are becoming stronger and more adaptable.

Graceful control: Take note of how in control you feel during each movement. Are you able to perform the exercises with a sense of grace and precision? This signifies an enhanced mind-body connection, allowing for more refined execution.

Increased Stability

Balance check: Pay attention to how steady you feel as you hold positions. Are you noticing a greater sense of balance and control? This is a promising sign that your muscles, especially those supporting your core, are growing stronger.

Duration of stability: Observe how long you can maintain a stable position. Are you able to hold certain exercises for a longer period of time compared to Day 1? This indicates improved muscle endurance and overall stability.

Less wobbling: Notice if you experience less wobbling or trembling during challenging poses. Are you able to maintain a more solid and controlled posture? This suggests that your muscles are adapting and becoming more resilient.

Confidence in movements: Reflect on how confident you feel in your movements. Are you approaching exercises with a greater sense of assurance? This newfound confidence is a testament to your growing physical strength and stability.

Strength and Endurance

Increased holding time: Pay attention to your ability to maintain positions. Are you finding it easier to hold exercises like wall squats or planks for longer durations? This indicates a significant improvement in both strength and muscular endurance.

Enhanced execution: Take note of how much stronger you feel during movements like wall push-ups or leg lifts. Are you able to execute these exercises with more control and power? This is a clear sign of increasing muscular strength.

Reduced fatigue: Assess how quickly you tire during exercises. Are you noticing less fatigue and greater staying power? Improved endurance is a surefire sign that your muscles are adapting and growing more resilient.

Greater repetition capacity: Pay attention to how many repetitions you can comfortably perform. Are you able to complete more reps compared to when you started? This shows that your muscles are becoming more conditioned and capable.

Flexibility

Increased range of motion: Take note of how freely you can move during exercises like wall angels or side leg lifts. Are you able to extend and flex with greater ease? This signifies an improvement in flexibility.

Reduced stiffness: Check if you experience less stiffness in your muscles and joints. Are you finding it easier to transition between positions? This is a positive sign that your body is becoming more supple.

Enhanced stretching capacity: Evaluate how deeply you can stretch during exercises like wall taps or single-leg wall squats. Are you able to reach further than before? This indicates that your muscles are becoming more pliable.

Smooth transitions: Pay attention to how smoothly you can transition between different movements. Are you able to flow from one exercise to another with greater fluidity? This suggests an improvement in overall flexibility.

Breath Awareness

Controlled breathing: Notice if your breath has become more controlled, especially during exercises like wall planks or leg lifts. Are you able to regulate the rhythm of your breath more effectively? This is a sign of improved breath awareness.

Synchronized movements: Observe if your breath is in sync with your movements. Are you able to coordinate your inhales and exhales seamlessly with exercises like wall push-ups or wall squats? This indicates a deeper connection between your mind and body.

Steady respiratory rate: Check if your breath remains steady and even, even during challenging exercises. Are you able to maintain a consistent pace of breathing? This suggests an enhanced level of breath control.

Mindful breathing: Assess if you're more mindful of your breath throughout your practice. Are you able to focus on the sensation of your breath entering and leaving your body? This signifies a heightened awareness of the mind-body connection.

Reduced Discomfort

Initial sensations: Pay attention to how your body feels at the start of each exercise. Are you noticing any areas of discomfort or tension? Take note of these sensations.

Progressive changes: As the days go by, check if there's a reduction in any discomfort you initially felt. Are you experiencing less strain or tension in those specific areas?

Improved ease: Assess whether you're finding it easier to move through the exercises without the same level of discomfort. Are you able to perform the movements with greater ease and fluidity?

Feedback loop: Use any discomfort as feedback. Is it a temporary response to a new movement, or is it indicative of an adjustment needed in your form or technique?

By keeping track of these aspects, you'll be able to gauge your progress in terms of reducing discomfort and increasing overall comfort in your Wall Pilates practice.

In this chapter, we embarked on a transformative journey in Wall Pilates, spanning a month-long program designed to forge a resilient and balanced mind-body connection. A strong foundation is highlighted as the linchpin of any successful fitness venture, providing stability, resilience, and a solid base for growth. Over the next 29 days, we delve deep into Wall Pilates, sculpting strength, nurturing flexibility, and fostering mental clarity.

KEY TAKEAWAYS

- **Foundation is key:** A solid foundation is vital for any successful fitness journey. It provides stability, resilience, and a base for growth.
- **Holistic growth:** Through Wall Pilates, we not only enhance physical strength but also cultivate a newfound sense of inner strength and mental clarity.
- **Structured progression:** The 29-day program introduces exercises in a carefully designed progression, building upon each other to create a harmonious and empowered you.
- **Measuring improvement:** It's important to track progress. Pay attention to aspects like ease of execution, increased stability, strength and endurance, flexibility, breath awareness, and reduced discomfort.
- **Balanced routine:** Each week has a specific focus, gradually intensifying the exercises while paying attention to increased ease in performing them.
- **Mind-body connection:** Wall Pilates not only nurtures physical strength but also fosters a deep connection between mind and body, promoting a holistic sense of well-being.

By following this well-organized program and closely monitoring your advancements, you are laying the foundation for a remarkable journey in Wall Pilates. Dedication and mindfulness are the keys to unlocking the full potential of this transformative experience.

Commitment to the structured regimen is essential. It demonstrates your determination to improve and allows you to reap the full benefits of the exercises. Consistency in practice helps strengthen not only your physical body but also your mental fortitude. As you progress, you will notice increased flexibility, improved core strength, and enhanced posture.

Being mindful throughout your Wall Pilates journey is equally crucial. It means paying attention to your body's signals, understanding its limitations, and respecting its needs. Mindfulness encourages you to perform each movement with precision and intention, maximizing the effectiveness of the exercises. It also fosters a deeper connection between your mind and body, promoting a sense of overall well-being.

Remember to celebrate your achievements along the way. Recognizing your progress, no matter how small, is a vital part of the journey. Each milestone, whether it's holding a posture longer or achieving greater flexibility, is a testament to your dedication and hard work. These celebrations serve as motivation to continue pushing forward towards becoming a stronger, more balanced version of yourself.

CONCLUSION

As you've stood against the wall, breathing with intention, you've not just strengthened muscles but awakened a deeper sense of self. With every squat and every push-up, you've woven a fabric of resilience and grace.

Throughout this journey, you've unlocked the transformative potential of Wall Pilates. You've discovered that it's more than just exercise; it's a holistic practice that bridges the gap between your mind and body. The mindful movements, the intentional breathwork, and the nurturing community—all these elements converge to elevate not only your physical strength but your mental resilience. Remember, progress is a path, not a destination. Each day and each session is a step toward a more harmonious union of your body and soul.

Before we part ways, I want to share a story with you. Meet Martha, someone who, just like you, embarked on a journey with Wall Pilates. At the outset, the wall presented itself as a formidable partner. Yet, day by day, Martha's persistence and mindful approach began to alter her perception. What was once a challenge evolved into a harmonious connection between herself, the wall, and her body.

In the confines of Wall Pilates, Martha unearthed more than physical strength; she uncovered a profound self-awareness. Her story stands as a living testament to the potency of steady commitment, mindfulness, and an unshakable faith in one's potential.

As you step onto your own path, remember that you're not venturing alone. You're joining a community of countless individuals who have embraced this transformative practice. Deep within, you hold the potential for greatness, and Wall Pilates is the fertile soil in which that potential can flourish.

Moving forward, let the walls be more than just support; let them be your canvas for self-discovery. Listen to your body, honor its wisdom, and let it guide you through each movement.

In the quiet spaces between breaths, in the strength of every muscle engagement, you've uncovered a sanctuary of stillness, a refuge from the chaos of the world. Carry this sanctuary with you, not just in your practice but in your daily life.

You've now delved into the principles, exercises, and power of community within Wall Pilates. The torch has been passed to you, ready for you to commence or advance on this path, fortifying not only your body but your mind as well. Seize the moment, take that first step, and revel in the multitude of benefits that Wall Pilates stands poised to bestow upon you.

This journey doesn't end here. It's a continuum of growth, a perpetual evolution. Keep exploring, keep listening, and keep moving. Your body is a symphony, and Wall Pilates is your conductor's baton. With every graceful movement, you're composing a masterpiece of health and well-being.

With every session, you're not just sculpting your physique; you're nurturing your soul. Remember, the power to transform is within you. You are your own beacon of strength and resilience.

If you found this book valuable on your journey through Wall Pilates, I would be grateful for your feedback. Your thoughts and experiences can inspire others on their own paths. Please take a moment to share your review. Thank you for being a part of this transformative journey!

Scan the QR code below to leave your review!

REFERENCES

Andersen, H. (2023, August 3). *Strengthen Your Core With Wall Pilates | New York Pilates*. Newyorkpilates.com. https://www.newyorkpilates.com/blog/wall-pilates-101/#:

Belanger, K. (n.d.). *Phyllis's Success Story. Improve Balance and Flexibility. Weight Loss*. Www.vintagefitness.ca. Retrieved October 17, 2023, from https://www.vintagefitness.ca/blog/2023/08/04/phyllis-success-story

BrainyQuote. (n.d.). *Les Brown Quotes*. BrainyQuote. https://www.brainyquote.com/quotes/les_brown_119176

Callicutt, S. (2020, June 24). *Why Should Senior Citizens Perform Balance Exercises?* Freedom Care. https://freedomcare.com/why-should-senior-citizens-perform-balance-exercises/

CDC. (2020, December 16). *Keep on Your Feet*. Centers for Disease Control and Prevention. https://www.cdc.gov/injury/features/older-adult-falls/index.html#:

Enterprise, S. to T. (2014, January 29). *Having good posture can improve your confidence, mood and overall health*. DavisEnterprise.com. https://www.davisenterprise.com/news/having-good-posture-can-improve-your-confidence-mood-and-overall-health/article_2b03d765-b514-5de5-b4d5-29576091b24e.html#:

Kendal at Home. (2023). *Eight (8) Simple Breathing Exercises for Older Adults*. Www.kendalathome.org. https://www.kendalathome.org/blog/breathe-easy-six-breath-exercises-for-older-adults

Kouvo, H. (2021, January 28). *Success story: Meet 2 "older" superwomen who prove the power of fitness | fitting fitness in*. Fitting Fitness In. https://www.fittingfitnessin.com/2021/01/success-story-meet-2-older-superwomen-who-prove-the-power-of-fitness/

Ohio State University. (2009, October 5). *Body Posture Affects Confidence In Your Own Thoughts, Study Finds*. ScienceDaily. https://www.sciencedaily.com/releases/2009/10/091005111627.htm

Orenstein, B. W. (2012, June 14). *How Fit Are You? A Fitness Test for Adults*. EverydayHealth.com. https://www.everydayhealth.com/fitness/how-fit-are-you-a-fitness-test-for-adults.aspx

Pilates Foundation. (2020). *The History of Pilates» Pilates Foundation*. Pilatesfoundation.com. https://www.pilatesfoundation.com/pilates/the-history-of-pilates/

Quinn, E. (2022, September 30). *Simple Tests to Measure Your Fitness Level at Home*. Verywell Fit. https://www.verywellfit.com/home-fitness-tests-3120282

Steers, S. (2020, January 31). *Pilates - One Man's Success Story*. Moving Spirit Pilates. https://movingspirit.ca/pilates-one-mans-success-story/

Ward, J. (2023, July 7). *The Power of Connections: Exploring the Mind-Body Connection and Building Relationships*. Burnalong. https://www.burnalong.com/blog/the-power-of-connections-exploring-the-mind-body-connection-and-building-relationships/#:

Made in the USA
Middletown, DE
22 August 2024

59595111R00102